QV77PUR

Drugs in Psychiatry

Drugs in Psychiatry

Second edition

Basant K. Puri

MA, PhD, MB, BChir, BSc (Hons) MathSci, FRCPsych,
DipStat, MMath, FSB
Hammersmith Hospital and Imperial College London, UK

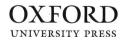

OXFORD
UNIVERSITY PRESS

OXFORD
UNIVERSITY PRESS

Great Clarendon Street, Oxford, OX2 6DP,
United Kingdom

Oxford University Press is a department of the University of Oxford.
It furthers the University's objective of excellence in research, scholarship,
and education by publishing worldwide. Oxford is a registered trade mark of
Oxford University Press in the UK and in certain other countries

British Library Cataloguing in Publication Data

Data available

Library of Congress Cataloging in Publication Data

Library of Congress Control Number: 2012945092

ISBN 978–0–19–967044–4

Printed in China by
C&C Offset Printing Co. Ltd

Preface to the Second Edition

Following the success of the first edition of this pocket-book, I am grateful to Oxford University Press for the opportunity to write a second edition. The number of chapters has been increased from 10 to 12, with the inclusion of new chapters on treatment-resistant schizophrenia and treatment-resistant depression. The chapter on the principles of psychopharmacology now includes an expanded section on central nervous system neurotransmitters. Other chapters have been updated to include relevant results of new research studies. There have been several new psychopharmacological agents introduced into clinical practice since the appearance of the first edition; these are included in the present edition.

BP
2012

Preface to the Second Edition

Preface to the First Edition

This pocket-book gives details of all the major drugs used in clinical psychiatric practice with which medical students, junior doctors, and general practitioners should be familiar. It starts by briefly discussing drugs in psychiatry, and then considers the principles of psychopharmacology, which form the foundation of the sound, scientifically-based use of drugs in psychiatry. Details are then given, in turn, of the main non-depot antipsychotic drugs, antipsychotic depot injections, antimanic drugs, tricyclic and related antidepressant drugs, monoamine-oxidase inhibitors, selective serotonin re-uptake inhibitors, and other antidepressants. Finally, the last chapter briefly describes other drugs used in psychiatry, including those which should only be initiated by specialists with expertise in certain areas of clinical practice.

BP
April 2006

Preface to the First Edition

Contents

Detailed Contents *xi*
Symbols and Abbreviations *xv*

1	Drug treatment and psychiatry	**1**
2	The principles of psychopharmacology	**11**
3	Non-depot antipsychotic drugs	**37**
4	Antipsychotic depot injections	**95**
5	Treatment-resistant schizophrenia	**111**
6	Antimanic drugs	**113**
7	Tricyclic and related antidepressant drugs	**135**
8	Monoamine-oxidase inhibitors	**155**
9	Selective serotonin re-uptake inhibitors	**169**
10	Other and newer antidepressant drugs	**189**
11	Treatment-resistant depression	**205**
12	Other drugs used in psychiatry	**207**

References *217*
Index *219*

Detailed Contents

Symbols and Abbreviations *xv*

1 Drug treatment and psychiatry   **1**
    The use of drugs in psychiatry *2*
    The nature of psychiatric disorders *3*
    The diagnostic hierarchical model in psychiatry *4*
    The need for a full assessment *6*

2 The principles of psychopharmacology   **11**
    Classification of psychotropic drugs *12*
    The principles of absorption, distribution, metabolism,
        and elimination of drugs *14*
    Pharmacokinetic terms and formulae *22*
    Pharmacokinetics in neonates and babies *30*
    Pharmacokinetics in the elderly *31*
    Drug receptors *32*
    Receptor superfamilies *33*
    Neurotransmitter systems *34*

3 Non-depot antipsychotic drugs   **37**
    Use of antipsychotic drugs *38*
    Classification of first-generation antipsychotic drugs *40*
    Second-generation antipsychotic drugs *42*
    NICE guidance *43*
    CATIE and CUtLASS *44*
    Equivalent doses *45*
    High doses *46*
    Overall cautions and contraindications *48*
    Withdrawal of antipsychotic drugs *50*
    Extrapyramidal symptoms *52*
    Neuroleptic malignant syndrome *54*
    Effects of antipsychotic drugs on brain structure *56*
    Elderly patients *58*
    Chlorpromazine *60*
    Trifluoperazine *62*
    Haloperidol *63*
    Pimozide *64*
    Flupentixol *66*
    Zuclopenthixol *68*
    Sulpiride *70*
    Second-generation antipsychotic drugs: side-effects
        and cautions *71*
    Amisulpride *72*
    Aripiprazole *74*
    Clozapine *76*

Olanzapine *80*
Paliperidone *84*
Quetiapine *86*
Risperidone *90*
Asenapine *93*

4 Antipsychotic depot injections   **95**
Administration *96*
Dosage guidelines *99*
Equivalent doses *100*
Choice *101*
Flupentixol decanoate *102*
Fluphenazine decanoate *103*
Haloperidol decanoate *104*
Olanzapine embonate *105*
Paliperidone *106*
Pipotiazine palmitate *107*
Risperidone *108*
Zuclopenthixol decanoate *109*

5 Treatment-resistant schizophrenia   **111**
Treatment-resistant schizophrenia *112*

6 Antimanic drugs   **113**
The use of antimanic drugs *114*
Treatment strategies for bipolar I disorder *115*
Lithium salts *116*
Carbamazepine *122*
Valproic acid *128*
Second-generation antipsychotics *130*
Asenapine *132*

7 Tricyclic and related antidepressant drugs   **135**
The use of tricyclic antidepressants *136*
Dosage *137*
Choice *138*
Withdrawal *140*
Driving and the use of machinery *141*
Amitriptyline *142*
Imipramine *145*
Trimipramine *146*
Dosulepin *147*
Clomipramine *148*
Lofepramine *149*
Nortriptyline *150*
Doxepin *151*
Trazodone *152*
Mianserin *153*

8 Monoamine-oxidase inhibitors 155
The use of MAOIs *156*
Choice *159*
Withdrawal *160*
Phenelzine *161*
Isocarboxazid *164*
Tranylcypromine *165*
Reversible MAOIs *166*
Moclobemide *167*

9 Selective serotonin re-uptake inhibitors 169
The use of SSRIs *170*
Risk of suicide or hostility *171*
Interactions with MAOIs *172*
Withdrawal reactions and dependency *173*
Side-effects of SSRIs *174*
Efficacy *176*
Fluvoxamine *177*
Fluoxetine *178*
Sertraline *180*
Paroxetine *182*
Citalopram *184*
Escitalopram *186*

10 Other and newer antidepressants 189
Agomelatine *190*
Duloxetine *192*
Flupentixol *195*
Mirtazapine *196*
Reboxetine *198*
Venlafaxine *200*
Tryptophan *204*

11 Treatment-resistant depression 205
Treatment-resistant depression *206*

12 Other drugs used in psychiatry 207
Benzodiazepines *208*
Non-benzodiazepine hypnotics *209*
Buspirone *210*
Beta-adrenoceptor blocking drugs *211*
Barbiturates *212*
Central nervous system stimulants *213*
Antimuscarinic drugs used in parkinsonism *214*
Drugs used in substance dependence *215*
Drugs for Alzheimer's disease *216*

Symbols and Abbreviations

℔	structure
⟴	receptor binding
♒	dose
☺	side-effects
5-HT	5-hydroxytryptamine (serotonin)
AChE	acetylcholine esterase
ADH	antidiuretic hormone
ADHD	attention-deficit hyperactivity disorder
AUC	area under the curve
AV	atrioventricular
COMT	catechol-O-methyltransferase
CSM	Committee on Safety of Medicines
DOPA	3,4-dihydroxyphenylalanine
DOPAC	dihydroxyphenylacetic acid
ECG	electrocardiogram
GABA	G-aminobutyric acid
GTP	guanosine triphosphate
HVA	homovanillic acid
MAO	monoamine oxidase
MAOI	monoamine oxidase inhibitor
MHPG	3-methoxy-4-hydroxyphenylglycol
NARI	noradrenaline re-uptake inhibitor
NICE	National Institute for Health and Clinical Excellence
RIMA	reversible inhibitors of monoamine oxidase A
SLE	systemic lupus erythematosus
SSRI	selective serotonin reuptake inhibitor
VMA	vanillyl mandelic acid

Chapter 1

Drug treatment and psychiatry

The use of drugs in psychiatry 2
The nature of psychiatric disorders 3
The diagnostic hierarchical model in psychiatry 4
The need for a full assessment 6

The use of drugs in psychiatry

Many of the original 20th-century drug treatments for psychiatric disorders, including attention-deficit hyperactivity disorder (ADHD), schizophrenia, depression, and bipolar mood disorder, were based on serendipitous findings. In the 21st century, we are able to develop psychiatric drugs in a more logical manner, on the basis of our preclinical or scientific understanding of these and other disorders from fields as diverse as molecular genetics, lipid neuroscience, and neurospectroscopy.

While this book concentrates on the major types of drug treatment in psychiatry, it should be borne in mind that psychopharmacological interventions constitute just one part of the treatment regimen that is appropriate for most disorders. Other treatments that should be considered, and with which drug treatment can be properly integrated, may include cognitive-behavioural therapy, psychodynamic psychotherapy, group psychotherapy, family therapy, marital therapy, sex therapy, art therapy, music therapy, occupational therapy, psychoeducation, social skills training, rehabilitation, phototherapy, and nutritional supplementation.

When drug therapy is opted for, due regard should be given to the underlying principles of psychopharmacology. These are summarized in Chapter 2.

The nature of psychiatric disorders

In general, most psychiatric disorders can be dichotomized into organic disorders, which are secondary to physical causes, and functional disorders. Clearly, since modern neuroscience does not believe in a mind–body (or mind–brain) duality, there is a sense in which materialist scientists should expect that all functional psychiatric disorders will eventually be discovered to be organic. For now, we may consider the major organic psychiatric disorders to consist of:

- The organic disorders proper, including:
  - mental disorders caused by a medical condition (such as an endocrinopathy or carcinoma)
  - dementias
  - organic amnesic syndrome not induced by alcohol or another psychoactive substance
  - delirium.
- Mental and behavioural disorders caused by psychoactive substance use, such as:
  - alcohol
  - opioids
  - amphetamine (amfetamine) or amphetamine-like substances
  - cannabinoids
  - sedatives or hypnotics
  - cocaine
  - other stimulants such as caffeine
  - hallucinogens
  - tobacco or nicotine
  - volatile solvents.

The functional psychiatric disorders are traditionally divided into:

- Psychoses, such as:
  - schizophrenia
  - mood (affective) disorders
  - schizoaffective (schizo-mood) disorders
  - delusional disorders.
- Neuroses, such as:
  - phobic anxiety disorders
  - other anxiety disorders
  - obsessive–compulsive disorder
  - adjustment disorders
  - dissociative (conversion) disorders
  - somatoform disorders.

The diagnostic hierarchical model in psychiatry

Fig. 1.1 is a representation of the hierarchical model used in psychiatric diagnosis. When making a diagnosis, the disorder at the higher or highest level takes precedence. For instance, if a patient suffering from chronic schizophrenia suffers from depressive symptoms, the primary diagnosis made is schizophrenia rather than a mood (affective) disorder.

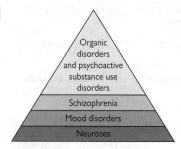

Fig. 1.1 Diagnostic hierarchy. (Reproduced with permission from Puri BK, Laking PJ, Treaseden IH (2003). *Textbook of Psychiatry*, 2nd edn. Churchill Livingstone, Edinburgh.)

The need for a full assessment

When treating psychiatric disorders, it is important to take a full history, carry out detailed mental state and physical examinations, and perform appropriate investigations. One reason for doing this is to ensure that your working diagnosis is accurate, so that you use the most appropriate treatment. The processes of history taking, mental state examination, physical examination, and investigations also can reveal key pieces of information that can be important when prescribing medication.

History

In the psychiatric history, the family history may reveal the possibility that the patient may be suffering from an inherited disease, such as an inherited liver disease (e.g. haemochromatosis and alpha-1 anti-trypsin deficiency), which in turn might be a contraindication for the drug of first choice. Another example relates to the inherited cytochrome P450 (CYP) 2C9 (CYP2C9) polymorphisms; genes encoding for R144C (*2) and I359L (*3) amino acid substitutions have relatively high population frequencies and may lead to pharmacokinetic effects. Pharmacogenetics-based dose adjustments may have to be made for certain drugs that are metabolized by the affected organ or enzyme isoform.

The occupational history may reveal that the patient operates machinery or has to drive for a living. It may be inadvisable to perform these activities while on certain types of medication, such as tricyclic antidepressants.

Other parts of the personal history may reveal that the patient is pregnant or breastfeeding; certain drugs are contraindicated or must be used with caution in pregnancy, while alternatives to breastfeeding may be appropriate for drugs that enter the breast milk and are likely to affect the baby.

The past medical history, current medication, and past psychiatric history may give an indication of the previous responses to different treatments, side-effects from drugs used, hypersensitivity reactions to drugs, and likely compliance with medication. Certain medical disorders are contraindications to treatment with certain drugs, while caution may need to be exercised with other drugs. For instance, second-generation antipsychotic (also known as atypical antipsychotic) medication should be used with caution in patients with cardiovascular disease or a history of epilepsy. The current medication also allows potential interactions with drugs being considered to be evaluated. For example, some psychotropic and antiepileptic drugs adversely affect the efficacy of oral contraception. Under the heading of current medication, it is important to take a history not just of prescribed drugs, but also those that are available over the counter (such as some analgesics and statins) and supplements (including herbal remedies). For instance, many depressed patients 'self-medicate' with St John's wort (*Hypericum perforatum*); St John's wort interferes with the cytochrome P450 monooxygenase system, increasing CYP3A4 activity and inhibiting CYP2D6. (Drugs that are contraindicated with St John's wort include carbamazepine, phenytoin, and selective serotonin reuptake inhibitors (SSRIs); the herbal remedy also impairs the action of oral contraceptives.)

The exploration of psychoactive substance use may point to the likelihood of hepatic impairment from alcohol abuse. As an example, in such a case, when choosing a traditional antidepressant, tricyclics might be preferred to traditional monoamine oxidase inhibitors (MAOIs), if the liver disease is not severe, although the sedative effects of the tricyclic antidepressants will be increased.

A forensic history of hostility or rage might lead to caution when considering the prescribing of benzodiazepines. The latter may cause disinhibition or dyscontrol reactions.

Mental state examination

The appearance and behaviour of the patient may show evidence of an endocrinopathy (such as hypothyroidism, hyperthyroidism, or Cushing's disease), Parkinson's disease, or parkinsonian side-effects. In turn, this may lead to caution in prescribing certain drugs (for instance, antipsychotic drugs should be used with caution in Parkinson's disease, which may be worsened by these drugs) or a decision to prescribe certain drugs (such as antimuscarinic medication for severe parkinsonian side-effects).

If the patient suffers from a needle phobia, then drug administration by injection should clearly be avoided if possible. The presence of suicidal and/or homicidal thoughts in a patient who self-administers their medication should point the prescriber towards drugs with a relatively wide therapeutic index (or indeed a non-pharmacological treatment option).

Rarely, a patient may be suffering from a delusion or overvalued idea relating to certain colours, shapes, letters, or names. In such cases, it is worth checking that the colour, shape, or name of tablets or capsules being prescribed are not likely to be misinterpreted by the patient.

Poor cognition and/or insight into the nature of his illness may be pointers to likely poor compliance by the patient. In such cases, alternatives to self-administration of oral medication may need to be considered; for instance, depot injections instead of oral antipsychotics, or supervised oral administration.

Physical examination

A full physical examination should routinely be carried out for a new patient or for a patient with the first presentation of a serious psychiatric illness. It is also good practice to do this in the case of the new onset of psychiatric symptoms, in treatment-resistant patients, or if there is anything from the history or mental state examination that suggests an organic disorder. Always bear in mind that the list of organic disorders that can present with psychiatric symptomatology is very long. To take one example, there have been too many cases of patients with primary hypoadrenalism (Addison's disease) being treated for years with antidepressant medication, until one day a doctor examines them and elicits signs compatible with the organic diagnosis but not with depression. Incidentally, in the presence of conditions associated with sodium ion imbalance such as Addison's disease, caution must be exercised in considering pharmacotherapy with lithium salts.

In the case of liver disease, psychotropic drugs that should be avoided or used with caution include:
• Acamprosate—should be avoided in severe liver disease.
• Antidepressants: MAOIs—idiosyncratic hepatotoxicity may result.

- Antidepressants: SSRIs and SSRI-like—these should be avoided altogether in severe hepatic disease, and should be used in lower doses, if at all, in less severe cases.
- Antidepressants: tricyclic and tricyclic-related—these should be avoided altogether in severe hepatic disease, while in less severe cases note that the sedative effects of these drugs may be increased.
- Antipsychotics—these can precipitate coma in liver disease; phenothiazine typical antipsychotic drugs are themselves hepatotoxic.
- Anxiolytics and hypnotics—these can precipitate coma in liver disease and should be avoided if possible; in cases of non-severe liver disease, if they have to be used, reduced doses of zaleplon (5mg maximum for an adult), zolpidem (5mg maximum for an adult), or zopiclone may be prescribed, while the *British National Formulary* recommends that if hypnotic treatment in a patient suffering from non-severe hepatic impairment is necessary, then a small dose of a benzodiazepine with a relatively short half-life, such as temazepam or oxazepam, may be considered (but benzodiazepines, zaleplon, zolpidem, and zopiclone should be *avoided* if there is severe hepatic impairment).
- Atomoxetine—reduced dosages need to be used if this drug for ADHD has to be prescribed; note that atomoxetine may itself cause hepatic impairment.
- Carbamazepine—its metabolism is impaired by hepatic disease.
- Cyproterone acetate—dose-related toxicity occurs.
- Modafinil—the dose should be halved in severe liver disease.
- Sodium valproate—see valproic acid.
- Valproate—see valproic acid.
- Valproic acid—should be avoided if possible; there is a risk of hepatotoxicity and hepatic failure (particularly during the first 6 months).

In the case of renal impairment, psychotropic drugs that should be avoided or used with caution include:
- Acamprosate—should be avoided in moderate to severe renal impairment.
- Antipsychotics—in general, reduced doses should be used; there is increased cerebral sensitivity in severe renal impairment.
- Anxiolytics and hypnotics—small doses should be used to begin with; there is increased cerebral sensitivity in severe renal impairment.
- Buspirone—a reduced dose should be used in mild renal impairment, while the drug should be avoided in moderate to severe renal impairment.
- Carbamazepine—caution should be exercised in prescribing this drug in renal impairment.
- Escitalopram—caution should be exercised in prescribing this drug in mild renal impairment.
- Fluoxetine—should be avoided in severe renal impairment; a reduced dose should be used in mild to moderate renal impairment, by giving the drug on alternate days.
- Fluvoxamine—in moderate renal impairment, a smaller starting dose should be used.

- Lithium salts—these should be avoided; in mild renal impairment, if lithium salts *have* to be used, the dose should be reduced and the plasma concentration monitored carefully.
- Mirtazapine—caution should be exercised in prescribing this drug in renal impairment.
- Modafinil—in severe renal impairment half the normal dose should be used.
- Sertraline—caution should be exercised in prescribing this drug in renal impairment.
- Sodium valproate—see valproic acid.
- Valproate—see valproic acid.
- Valproic acid—the dose should be reduced.
- Venlafaxine—if the creatinine clearance is between 10–30mL/minute, half the normal dose of venlafaxine should be used; if the creatinine clearance is less than 10mL/minute, venlafaxine should be avoided.

Investigations

An important type of investigation is gleaning further information from relatives, the patient's general practitioner, and from other professionals involved in the case. First-line physical investigations include a full blood count, urea and electrolytes, thyroid function tests, liver function tests, vitamin B12 and folate levels, and syphilis serology. These may reveal the presence of an endocrinopathy, a metabolic disturbance, or hepatic impairment, for example. Second-line investigations, such as the creatinine clearance, urinary drug screening, electroencephalography, neuropsychological testing, neuroimaging, and genetic tests, may be indicated by the history and examination.

Certain investigations should be carried out in association with the prescribing of specific psychotropic drugs. In the case of the intended prescription of antipsychotic drugs in doses higher than those recommended by the *British National Formulary*, the Royal College of Psychiatrists recommends (see Chapter 3) that an electrocardiogram (ECG) be carried out to exclude untoward abnormalities such as a prolonged QT interval; the ECG should be repeated periodically and the antipsychotic dose should be reduced if there is a prolonged QT interval or another adverse ECG abnormality.

Before starting antipsychotic pharmacotherapy with clozapine, the leucocyte and differential blood counts need to be in the normal range. As clozapine can cause neutropenia and potentially fatal agranulocytosis, leucocyte and differential blood counts need to be monitored weekly for 18 weeks and then at least fortnightly. If treatment with clozapine is continued and the blood count remains stable after 1 year, then the leucocyte and differential blood counts should be monitored at least every 4 weeks. They should also be monitored 4 weeks following discontinuation of clozapine. Further details are given in Chapter 3.

It is good practice to check the white blood count in patients before starting treatment with olanzapine, as this antipsychotic drug should be used with caution in patients with a low leucocyte or neutrophil count.

Liver function tests should be carried out before starting treatment with valproic acid (as the semisodium salt), and should be monitored during at least the first 6 months of treatment.

Blood counts, hepatic and renal tests are recommended by the manufacturer when treating with carbamazepine.

Since lithium cations are excreted mainly by the kidneys, it is important to check a patient's renal function before commencing treatment with a lithium salt (see Chapter 6). It is also prudent to obtain baseline measures of the thyroid function tests, as thyroid function disturbances may result from long-term lithium therapy. Other blood test monitoring that should be carried out during lithium therapy is described in Chapter 6.

The principles of psychopharmacology

Classification of psychotropic drugs *12*
The principles of absorption, distribution, metabolism,
   and elimination of drugs *14*
Pharmacokinetic terms and formulae *22*
Pharmacokinetics in neonates and babies *30*
Pharmacokinetics in the elderly *31*
Drug receptors *32*
Receptor superfamilies *33*
Neurotransmitter systems *34*

Classification of psychotropic drugs

The classification of psychotropic drugs followed in this book is similar to that used by the *British National Formulary*. It is given together with the relevant chapter numbers from this book.

- Antipsychotic drugs:
  - non-depot antipsychotics (typical, e.g. chlorpromazine, and atypical, e.g. aripiprazole) (Chapter 3)
  - depot antipsychotics, e.g. flupentixol decanoate (Chapter 4).
- Antimanic drugs—e.g. lithium salts, carbamazepine, and valproic acid (Chapter 6).
- Antidepressants:
  - tricyclic and related antidepressants, e.g. amitriptyline (Chapter 7)
  - monoamine-oxidase inhibitors, e.g. moclobemide (Chapter 8)
  - selective serotonin re-uptake inhibitors, e.g. escitalopram (Chapter 9)
  - other antidepressants, e.g. agomelatine (Chapter 10).
- Hypnotics—e.g. zaleplon (Chapter 12).
- Anxiolytics—e.g. lorazepam (Chapter 12).
- Barbiturates (Chapter 12).
- Central nervous system stimulants—e.g. atomoxetine (Chapter 12).
- Antimuscarinic drugs used in parkinsonism—e.g. procyclidine (Chapter 12).
- Drugs used in substance dependence—e.g. acamprosate (Chapter 12).
- Drugs for dementia—e.g. memantine (Chapter 12).

The principles of absorption, distribution, metabolism, and elimination of drugs

When a psychotropic drug is administered to a patient, the pharmacokinetic processes relating to the drug refer to the effects of his body on the actions of this medication and include the processes of its absorption, distribution, metabolism and elimination. For most drugs, systemic circulation drug concentration is related to drug concentration at its sites of action, as shown in Fig. 2.1. By knowing the pharmacokinetics of a drug, together with the drug dose taken, it is possible to calculate drug concentration as a function of time at the sites of drug action.

Absorption

The processes by means of which a drug leaves its site of administration and enters the systemic circulation are referred to as drug absorption. The main types of absorption can be classified as follows:
- Enteral administration—drug absorption into the systemic circulation from the gastrointestinal tract:
  - oral
  - buccal or sublingual
  - rectal.
- Parenteral administration—drug absorption into the systemic circulation from sites other than the gastrointestinal tract:
  - intramuscular
  - intravenous
  - subcutaneous
  - inhalational
  - topical
  - intranasal
  - intra-arterial
  - intrathecal.

Factors which affect the rate of drug absorption include:
- The form of the drug:
  - enteric coating, for example, slows down drug disintegration in the stomach.
- The solubility of the drug, which depends on:
  - the pK_a of the drug, which is the pH at which precisely half of the drug is in its ionized form
  - the size of particles in the formulation
  - the pH.
- The rate of blood flow at the site of administration:
  - the higher the blood flow, the greater the rate of drug absorption.

Distribution

The distribution of a drug follows its absorption, or direct administration, into the systemic blood circulation and refers to the way in which it is

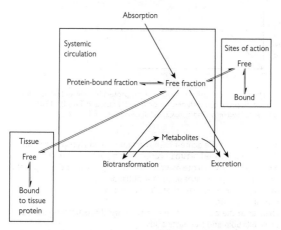

Fig. 2.1 The relationship between drug pharmacokinetics and the concentration of the drug in the systemic circulation and at its sites of action.

distributed between the lipid, protein, and water compartments. Factors which influence drug distribution include the following:
- Haemodynamic factors:
  - cardiac output.
  - regional blood flow—those organs with the highest blood perfusion rates, such as (under normal circumstances) the brain, liver, and kidneys, receive the highest distribution to begin with, while a second distribution phase then gradually sees a redistribution to tissues such as resting skeletal muscle, adipose tissue, most viscera and the skin.
- Plasma-protein binding. This acts as a drug reservoir since pharmacological activity, if it exists, resides with the free (unbound) drug fraction. As shown in Fig. 2.1, the free fraction and the protein-bound fraction are in equilibrium with each other. Acidic drugs mainly bind to albumin. Many psychotropic drugs are basic, and they may bind to, for example, α_1-acid glycoprotein and lipoprotein. Plasma-protein binding is usually reversible (not covalent). Factors that can alter the degree of plasma-protein binding include:
  - plasma drug concentration—the usual relationship between plasma-protein binding and plasma drug concentration is that shown in Fig. 2.2
  - hypoalbuminaemia—for instance as a result of hepatic or renal disease, cardiac failure, malnutrition, carcinoma, surgery, or burns
  - acute phase response—disorders causing this, including myocardial infarction, carcinoma, arthritis, and Crohn's disease, can raise the

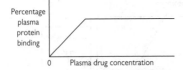

Fig. 2.2 The usual relationship between plasma-protein binding and plasma drug concentration. Reproduced with permission from Puri BK and Tyer PJ (1998). *Sciences Basic to Psychiatry*, 2nd edn. Churchill Livingstone, Edinburgh.

   plasma level of the acute-phase reactant α_1-acid glycoprotein (and therefore increased plasma-protein binding of basic drugs)
   • hypo-α_1-acid glycoproteinaemia—which may occur in the nephrotic syndrome, hepatic disease and malnutrition
   • hyperlipoproteinaemia—types IIa, IIb, and IV
   • drug interaction
   • changes in the concentration of physiological substances—such as urea, bilirubin and free fatty acids.
• Permeability factors. In general, the higher the lipid-solubility of a drug, the greater its rate of entry into cells.
• The blood–brain barrier. This acts as a functional barrier between the cerebral circulation and the brain and is formed from:
   • the tight junctions between adjacent endothelial cells
   • the gliovascular membrane (formed from astrocytic perivascular feet on capillaries)
   • the capillary basement membrane
   • membrane transporters acting as efflux carriers—particularly P-glycoprotein.
• In general, the higher the lipid-solubility of a drug, the greater the probability that it will cross the blood–brain barrier. The blood–brain barrier may have altered properties in the presence of infection. (For instance, while normally penicillins, being highly water-soluble, do not readily cross the blood–brain barrier, during acute bacterial meningitis this situation changes markedly.) Active transport mechanisms are used to gain entry into the central nervous system by certain substances, such as levodopa. Note that small molecules (e.g. lithium ions) tend to be able to diffuse into the brain (and cerebrospinal fluid) from the systemic circulation.
• The blood–cerebrospinal fluid barrier. This is similar to the blood–brain barrier and exists at the choroid plexus. The tight junctions in the blood–cerebrospinal fluid barrier are between adjacent epithelial cells (as opposed to adjacent endothelial cells in the case of the blood–brain barrier).
• The placenta. Drug transfer across the placenta from the maternal circulation to the fetal circulation may take place via:
   • passive diffusion
   • active transport
   • pinocytosis.

- In general, it should be assumed that there is fetal exposure to any drugs or food supplements taken by the mother during pregnancy. Placental drug transfer is of importance throughout pregnancy owing the distinct possibility of adverse effects on the growing fetus or baby:
  - first trimester—teratogenesis may result (the highest risk period is between the 3rd and 11th weeks). If possible, all drugs and food supplements should be avoided during the first trimester. If a drug has to be given during this time, the smallest effective dose should be used and preference should be given to using a drug that has a history of having been used apparently safely in pregnancy rather than a newer drug or a drug that has no well-established history of safe use during pregnancy.
  - second and third trimesters—drugs may affect fetal growth and development. Toxic side-effects may occur in fetal tissues.
  - parturition—drugs given during labour may affect the neonate.

Metabolism

The metabolism or biotransformation of a drug generally renders it less lipid-soluble and more water-soluble. The products of such metabolism are more readily eliminated from the body. These products are not necessarily pharmacologically inactive. For instance, the serotonin re-uptake inhibitor fluoxetine is metabolized to the active drug norfluoxetine, while the benzodiazepine diazepam is metabolized to the active drug nordiazepam. Similarly, paliperidone (9-hydroxyrisperidone) is an active metabolite of risperidone.

Some highly water-soluble drugs, such as lithium salts, are excreted unchanged by the body.

The major site of drug metabolism is the liver. Other sites of significant biotransformation (which probably occurs in all tissues) are the:

- gastrointestinal tract
- kidneys
- lungs
- suprarenal (adrenal) cortex
- placenta
- skin
- lymphocytes.

Two phases are broadly defined for hepatic biotransformation, as shown in Fig. 2.3.

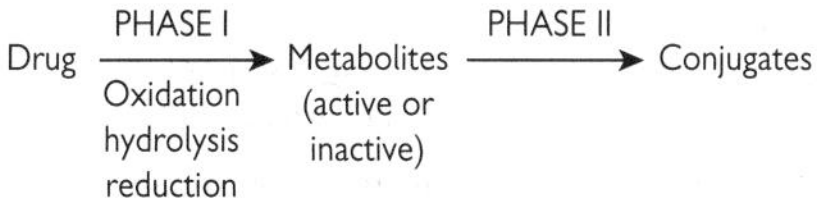

Drug $\xrightarrow[\substack{\text{Oxidation}\\\text{hydrolysis}\\\text{reduction}}]{\text{PHASE I}}$ Metabolites (active or inactive) $\xrightarrow{\text{PHASE II}}$ Conjugates

Fig. 2.3 Phase I and phase II metabolism (biotransformation). Reproduced with permission from Puri BK and Tyer PJ (1998). *Sciences Basic to Psychiatry*, 2nd edn. Churchill Livingstone, Edinburgh.

Phase I metabolism causes molecular structure changes by means of one or more of the following non-synthetic reactions:

- Oxidation—by microsomal mixed-function oxidases using the cytochrome P450 monooxygenase system, particularly CYP3A4, CYP3A5, CYP2C, and CYP2D6. Oxidative reactions and examples of drugs metabolized by them include:
  - aliphatic hydroxylation—e.g. meprobamate, pentobarbital
  - aromatic hydroxylation—e.g. amphetamine, phenytoin, propranolol
  - N-dealkylation (N-demethylation)—e.g. diazepam, amitriptyline, imipramine
  - O-dealkylation (O-demethylation)—e.g. codeine
  - S-dealkylation (S-demethylation)—e.g. 6-methyl thiopurine
  - deamination—e.g. amphetamine, diazepam
  - S-oxidation—e.g. chlorpromazine
  - Epoxidation—e.g. carbamazepine, phenytoin.
- Hydrolysis—in the smooth endoplasmic reticulum; it is not a common phase I reaction (e.g. pethidine).
- Reduction—in the smooth endoplasmic reticulum; it is not a common phase I reaction.

A drug or drug metabolite (from a phase I reaction) is conjugated to a polar (water-soluble) group by phase II metabolism. The result is a water-soluble conjugate which can undergo renal excretion relatively easily if it has a relative molecular mass (molecular weight) of less than approximately 300. If the relative molecular mass is much higher than 300, excretion can occur via the bile.

Conjugation reactions and examples of corresponding drug substrates include conjugation with:

- glucuronic acid—e.g. lorazepam, oxazepam, phenytoin
- sulphate—e.g. estrone
- acetate—e.g. hydralazine
- glutathione—e.g. metabolites such as epoxides
- glycine—e.g. salicylates.

Phase I and phase II metabolic enzyme activity may be increased by certain drugs. In turn, this can result in increased metabolism of these drugs themselves and/or other drugs. Examples of drugs that cause enzyme induction include:

- alcohol (ethanol)—induces increased metabolism of alcohol, barbiturates, bilirubin, meprobamate and phenytoin
- barbiturates—induce increased metabolism of barbiturates, chlorpromazine, the oral contraceptive pill, phenytoin, tricyclic antidepressants, etc.
- carbamazepine—induces increased metabolism of carbamazepine
- phenothiazines—induce increased metabolism of phenothiazines.

Note that enzyme induction does not necessarily reduce the risk of adverse side-effects. For example, microsomal enzyme induction by chronic alcohol (ethanol) intake can lead to increased levels of potentially hepatotoxic paracetamol phase I metabolites.

Drug metabolism that an orally administered drug undergoes by the liver or gut wall before entry into the systemic circulation is the first-pass effect (also known as first-pass metabolism, first-pass elimination, pre-systemic metabolism, and presystemic elimination). The result can be a substantial reduction in drug bioavailability, so that a higher oral dose needs to be given. Furthermore, there may be a high degree of variation in the level of the first-pass effect between different individuals.

Examples of drugs which undergo a high degree of first-pass metabolism include:
• imipramine—only 30–80% of the oral dose enters the systemic circulation intact
• fluphenazine—only around 10% of the oral dose enters the systemic circulation intact.

The level of the first-pass effect may be reduced in a number of ways:
• increased hepatic blood flow—following the ingestion of food or after taking a drug such as hydralazine
• hepatic impairment—e.g. as a result of hepatic cirrhosis.

Elimination

The major organ of drug excretion is the kidney. Drug excretion can also occur though:
• bile and faeces
• lungs
• saliva
• sweat
• sebum
• tears
• milk.

The key processes involved in the renal excretion of drugs are:
• Glomerular filtration. This amount of drug that enters the glomerular filtrate depends on factors such as the:
  • glomerular filtration rate
  • plasma water drug concentration
  • relative molecular mass of the drug.
• Active tubular secretion from the plasma to the glomerular filtrate of charged molecules in the proximal renal tubule. There are 2 main systems, for:
  • organic acids—e.g. glucuronide drug metabolites
  • organic bases—e.g. amphetamine.
• Passive tubular reabsorption from the glomerular filtrate to the blood, since the former becomes increasingly concentrated as it passes along the nephron. The extent of this reabsorption varies with drug/metabolite lipid solubility, which in turn varies with the:
  • pK_a of the drug or metabolite
  • pH of the tubular urine—e.g. reduced reabsorption occurs in alkaline tubular urine of acidic drugs, hence the use of forced alkaline diuresis in cases of aspirin (salicylate) and phenobarbitone overdose.

Conditions causing reduced renal clearance (e.g. renal disease) can reduce the excretion of drugs such as lithium salts, thereby resulting in lithium toxicity.

Cycling processes are processes in which, following excretion, some drugs may be reabsorbed into the systemic circulation, thereby being recycled. Examples of cycling processes include:

• the enterohepatic cycle—reabsorption of a drug (or drug metabolite) from the intestinal tract following hepatic excretion in bile
• gastric excretion—reabsorption of a drug (or drug metabolite) from the intestinal tract following gastric excretion
• salivary excretion—reabsorption of a drug (or drug metabolite) from the intestinal tract following salivary excretion.

Pharmacokinetic terms and formulae

Volume of distribution

This theoretical entity is the quotient of the drug dose (or drug mass), D, in the body to the plasma or blood concentration, C, of the drug at that time. The volume of distribution, V_d, is given by:

$$V_d = D/C \qquad \text{(Equation 2.1)}$$

Therefore the volume of distribution is the theoretical blood or plasma volume needed to account for the drug dose taken, to give the measured drug concentration. The volume of distribution does not usually correspond to either an anatomical or a physiological volume.

Half-life

Following intravenous injection, there is a rapid fall in the plasma drug concentration. This is caused by redistribution of the drug from the blood circulation into other tissues. The time taken for this redistribution process to halve the initial peak drug concentration is the distribution half-life, as shown in Fig. 2.4. As indicated in this diagram, the redistribution process is usually a rapid process, with a correspondingly short half-life.

Following redistribution, the slower process of drug elimination becomes increasingly evident. The time taken by this elimination process to halve the plasma drug concentration is the elimination half-life, also shown in Fig. 2.4.

Suppose a drug were being administered by continuous intravenous infusion. If the plasma concentration of the drug reached a constant value of C_0, and if the elimination half-life were constant at $t_{1/2}$, then, ignoring any redistribution effects, upon suddenly stopping the infusion (at time zero) the plasma drug concentrations at integer (whole number) multiples of the half-life would be as shown in Table 2.1.

Clearance

The clearance, Cl, of a drug is the volume of biological fluid (e.g. blood or plasma) which is cleared of the drug in unit time. The clearance is directly proportional to the volume of distribution:

$$Cl = k\, V_d \qquad \text{(Equation 2.2)}$$

where the constant of proportionality, k, is the first-order elimination constant, described later.

The clearance of a drug is also equivalent to the total rate of elimination of the drug with respect to the drug concentration, C, in a given biological fluid:

$$Cl = \text{total rate of elimination}/C \qquad \text{(Equation 2.3)}$$

The relationship of the drug clearance to the drug's elimination half-life, $t_{1/2}$, is given by:

$$Cl = (V_d \ln 2)/t_{1/2} \qquad \text{(Equation 2.4)}$$

in which ln 2 is the natural logarithm of 2 ($\log_e 2$) and is an irrational number equal to 0.69314718055994530941723212145818…

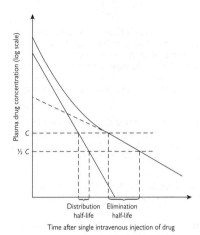

Fig. 2.4 A graph of the logarithm of the plasma drug concentration versus the time elapsing following one intravenous injection of the drug. The distribution and elimination half-lives are shown.

Table 2.1 The plasma drug concentration as a function of its elimination half-life, $t_{1/2}$. Adapted with permission from Puri BK and Tyer PJ (1998). *Sciences Basic to Psychiatry*, 2nd edn. Churchill Livingstone, Edinburgh.

Time	Plasma concentration
Zero	C_0
$t_{1/2}$	$C_0/2$
$2t_{1/2}$	$C_0/4$
$3t_{1/2}$	$C_0/8$
$4t_{1/2}$	$C_0/16$
$5t_{1/2}$	$C_0/32$
.	
.	
.	.
.	
$nt_{1/2}$	$C_0/2^n$

The total clearance is the sum of the clearances of the drug by all organs that eliminate that drug:

$$Cl = Cl_{renal} + Cl_{hepatic} + \ldots \qquad \text{(Equation 2.5)}$$

Bioavailability

The bioavailability of a drug is the fraction, F, of the administered drug dose which circumvents the first-pass effect (see p.19) and actually reaches the systemic circulation. At one extreme, when the whole drug dose reaches the systemic circulation, F takes the value one. At the other extreme, when none of the administered dose reaches the systemic circulation, F takes the value zero. Therefore, the range of values taken by the bioavailability is given by:

$$0 \leq F \leq 1 \qquad \text{(Equation 2.6)}$$

When the plasma drug concentration is plotted against time, as in Fig. 2.4, the area under the curve (AUC) is directly proportional to the amount of the drug which enters the systemic circulation. If a drug is administered by a non-intravenous route, then its bioavailability can be calculated using the following expression:

F = (AUC following administration by a given route)/(AUC following intravenous administration of the same dose)   (Equation 2.7)

First-order elimination

First-order elimination is also referred to as linear kinetics and occurs when the rate of drug elimination is directly proportional to its plasma concentration, C. Expressed using the differential calculus, this means that the rate of change of the plasma concentration is given by:

$$dC/dt = -kC \qquad \text{(Equation 2.8)}$$

where k is the first-order elimination constant, as mentioned earlier, and has a positive value. The minus sign occurs on the right-hand side of Equation 2.8 because for higher drug concentrations the rate of change of drug concentration is lower than for lower concentrations. It follows from Equation 2.8 that

$$\ln (C_0/2) = \ln C_0 - kt_{1/2} \qquad \text{(Equation 2.9)}$$

where, as before, $t_{1/2}$ is the elimination half-life of the drug.

From Equation 2.9 it follows that the drug's elimination half-life is given by:

$$t_{1/2} = (\ln 2)/k \qquad \text{(Equation 2.10)}$$

Since k and $\ln 2$ are constants, it follows that in first-order elimination the elimination half-life of a drug is constant.

Zero-order elimination

Zero-order elimination is also referred to as saturation kinetics and occurs when the rate of drug elimination is constant (and therefore independent of its plasma concentration, C). This can occur when, after reaching a certain threshold concentration, the enzyme(s) involved in drug elimination become saturated. A common example in psychiatric practice of a drug which is subject to zero-order elimination is ethanol (ethyl alcohol), at least when its plasma concentration exceeds around 0.1mg/mL.

Intravenous injection

If it is assumed that, following intravenous injection of a drug, it dissolves in one compartment (the one-compartment model), then, if drug clearance from that compartment takes place via first-order elimination, then the relationship between the plasma drug concentration, C, and time, t, is given by:

$$\ln C = C_0 - kt \qquad \text{(Equation 2.11)}$$

where C_0 is the initial drug concentration following injection, that is, the concentration at time zero, and k is the first-order elimination constant. From Equation 2.11 it follows that a plot of the logarithm (to any base) of drug concentration against time will yield a straight line graph with gradient $-k$ (that is, a negative gradient, since k is a positive constant), and intercept on the vertical axis (ordinate) of C_0. This is shown in Fig. 2.5. This means that the value of the elimination constant can be readily calculated from the gradient of such a line.

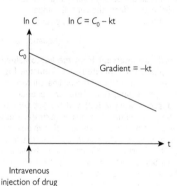

Fig. 2.5 One-compartment model for a single intravenous injection of a drug which undergoes first-order elimination. Adapted with permission from Puri BK and Tyer PJ (1998). *Sciences Basic to Psychiatry*, 2nd edn. Churchill Livingstone, Edinburgh.

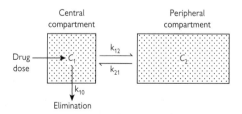

Fig. 2.6 Two-compartment model, in which the drug concentration in the central compartment is denoted by C_1 and the drug concentration in the peripheral compartment by C_2. Adapted with permission from Puri BK and Tyer PJ (1998). *Sciences Basic to Psychiatry*, 2nd edn. Churchill Livingstone, Edinburgh.

In general, the pharmacokinetics of drugs used in psychiatry tend to be better modelled by a two-compartment model, as shown in Fig. 2.6. Here, there are three constants:

- k_{10}—the first-order elimination constant
- k_{12}—the first-order rate constant for drug transfer from the central compartment to the peripheral compartment
- k_{21}—the first-order rate constant for drug transfer from the peripheral compartment to the central compartment.

A plot of the logarithm of the drug concentration against time for the two-compartment model, following a single intravenous drug injection, is as shown in Fig. 2.4. The fall in plasma drug concentration follows two phases. The first phase, corresponding to drug distribution (from the central systemic circulation compartment to the peripheral compartment), has gradient that is steeper (in an absolute sense) than that of the second phase, corresponding to drug elimination (from the central compartment). The drug concentration in the central compartment, C_1, is given by:

$$C_1 = Ae^{-\alpha t} + Be^{-\beta t} \qquad \text{(Equation 2.12)}$$

where A is the value of the ordinate intercept from the line obtained by subtracting the elimination phase (extrapolated) line from the log-plasma concentration-time curve, B is the value of the ordinate intercept of the extrapolated elimination phase line, α is minus the product of the natural logarithm of 10 (approximately 2.303) and the gradient of the line obtained by subtracting the elimination phase (extrapolated) line from the log-plasma concentration-time curve, and β is minus the product of the natural logarithm of 10 and the gradient of the (extrapolated) elimination phase line. The constant ln 10 appears in the values of the gradients of the two lines because the graph in Fig. 2.4 is plotting the logarithm to base 10 of the central compartment drug concentration ($\log_{10} C_1$) against time, rather than the natural logarithm (ln C_1) against time.

Constant intravenous infusion

When a drug is being given by constant intravenous infusion, if it follows first-order elimination, then the ratio of the plasma drug concentration, C, at any given time t, to the steady-state drug plasma concentration, C_{ss}, is given by

$$C/C_{ss} = 1 - e^{-kt} \qquad \text{(Equation 2.13)}$$

From Equation 2.10 it can be seen that the elimination rate constant, k, has the value

$$k = (\ln 2)/t_{\frac{1}{2}} \qquad \text{(Equation 2.14)}$$

Hence Equation 2.13 tells us that the rate at which the plasma concentration reaches the steady-state concentration depends only on the drug's half-life. This is illustrated in Table 2.2.

Table 2.2 The percentage of the plasma steady-state drug concentration attained by a drug being administered by intravenous infusion at a constant rate and following first-order elimination. Adapted with permission from Puri BK and Tyer PJ (1998). *Sciences Basic to Psychiatry*, 2nd edn. Churchill Livingstone, Edinburgh.

Percentage of C_{ss} reached	Time taken
50	$t_{1/2}$
75	$2t_{1/2}$
88	$3t_{1/2}$
94	$4t_{1/2}$
97	$5t_{1/2}$

Multiple dosing

If a drug with bioavailability F is administered (not necessarily intravenously) at a dose D at a regular interval, T, then if the drug is subject to first-order elimination, for a one-compartment model the average steady-state plasma drug concentration C_{ss} is given by

$$C_{ss} = Dt_{1/2}F/(V_d T \ln 2) \qquad \text{(Equation 2.15)}$$

Furthermore, the ratio of the maximum plasma drug concentration, C_{max}, to the minimum plasma drug concentration, C_{min}, is given by

$$C_{max}/C_{min} = 2T/t_{1/2} \qquad \text{(Equation 2.16)}$$

Administering an initial loading dose allows the average steady-state plasma drug concentration to be achieved sooner, as shown in Fig. 2.7.

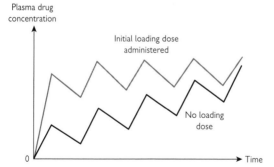

Fig. 2.7 The effect of administering an initial loading dose on the plasma drug concentration in the case of a drug being given at regular intervals. Adapted with permission from Puri BK and Tyer PJ (1998). *Sciences Basic to Psychiatry*, 2nd edn. Churchill Livingstone, Edinburgh.

Reducing the dosing interval leads to an increase in the average steady-state plasma drug concentration, as shown in Fig 2.8.

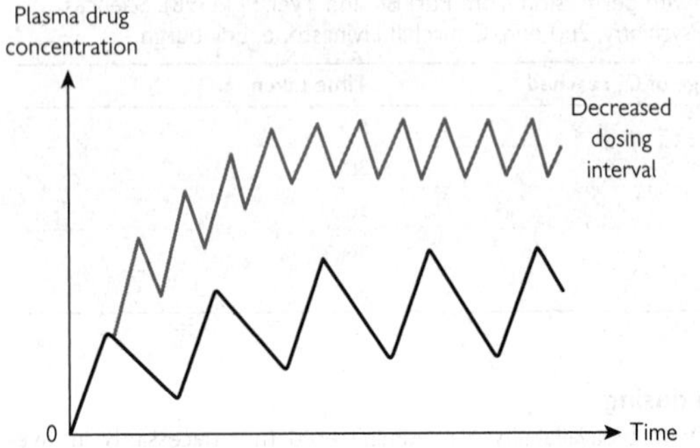

Fig. 2.8 The effect of reducing the dosing interval on the plasma drug concentration in the case of a drug being given at regular intervals. Adapted with permission from Puri BK and Tyer PJ (1998). *Sciences Basic to Psychiatry*, 2nd edn. Churchill Livingstone, Edinburgh.

Pharmacokinetics in neonates and babies

There are several considerations to bear in mind in respect of young humans compared with adults aged between 20–60 years:

- Neonates have a higher proportion of total body water.
- Neonates have a higher proportion of extracellular body water.
- Neonates have a lower proportion of adipose tissue.
- Neonates have a lower plasma concentration of albumin.
- Neonates have lower gastric acidity.
- Neonates have an increased gastric emptying time.
- Neonates have a more permeable blood–brain barrier.
- The glomerular filtration rate is lower in those aged less than 3–5 months.
- The microsomal enzyme activity in the liver is lower in those aged less than 2 months.

Pharmacokinetics in the elderly

Compared with younger adults, it is important to bear in mind that, in general, the elderly have:

- A reduced total body mass.
- A reduced proportion of total body water.
- A reduced proportion of muscle tissue.
- An increased proportion of adipose tissue.
- Different plasma concentrations of proteins—often a reduced level of plasma albumin and an increased level of plasma gamma-globulin, for example.
- Reduced hepatic metabolism.
- Reduced glomerular filtration rate.
- Reduced renal clearance.

Drug receptors

On binding to receptors, drugs can have various actions:
- Agonist—drug binding simulates the action of the receptor's endogenous ligand(s).
- Antagonist—drug binding does not have a stimulatory action and blocks the binding to the receptor of its endogenous agonist ligand(s).
- Partial agonist—the drug acts only partly as an agonist, without full agonist activity in spite of how high a dose is used.
- Inverse agonist—drug binding causes the receptor to be stabilized in a non-active state.

Dose-response curves showing some of these types of agonism appear in Fig. 2.9.

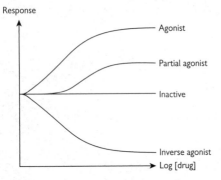

Fig. 2.9 Dose-response curves showing different types of agonism.

Receptor superfamilies

Several receptor superfamilies are now recognized, including the following.

G protein-coupled receptors

These involve guanosine triphosphate (GTP)-binding regulatory proteins. Second messengers that are regulated by drug/ligand-receptor binding include cAMP, cGMP, IP3, Ca^{2+}, and diacylglycerol. Many different drugs act on G protein-coupled receptors, as do large numbers of endogenous ligands, such as eicosanoids and the neurotransmitters acetylcholine, dopamine, noradrenaline (norepinephrine), serotonin, and opioid endorphins. In turn, many drugs used in psychiatry act on these neurotransmitters.

Cytoplasmic second messengers

The second messengers themselves may be the target of drug action. For instance, the antipsychotic chlorpromazine inhibits calmodulin, a calcium-modulated protein to which Ca^{2+} ions can bind.

Ion channels

There are many different ion channels, such as voltage-gated sodium ion channels and ligand-gated muscarinic acetylcholine M_2 receptors. Endogenous ligands include acetylcholine, several amino acids, the amino acid derivative γ-aminobutyric acid (GABA), and serotonin. An example of a drug class acting at such a receptor are the benzodiazepines, the binding of which to $GABA_A$ receptors lead to an increased inward flux of chloride ions.

Enzymes

Some receptors act as enzymes and may regulate the levels of neurotransmitters. Examples of such enzymes are monoamine oxidase (MAO) and acetylcholine esterase (AChE); drugs acting on these enzymes are used in clinical psychiatric practice—for instance, monoamine oxidase inhibitors (MAOIs) are used as antidepressants, while reversible inhibitors of AChE are used in the pharmacotherapy of Alzheimer's disease.

Nuclear transcription regulating receptors

These are involved in changes in gene transcription. Ligands include hormones such as sex hormones and thyroid hormone.

Carrier (transport) proteins

These carry out cell membrane transfer of small molecules across concentration gradients, as in the case of some neurotransmitters. One example is the protein DAT, which transports dopamine molecules. The anti-ADHD drug methylphenidate inhibits presynaptic re-uptake of dopamine by antagonizing the action of DAT.

Transmembrane non-enzyme receptors

These include cytokine receptors, for which cytokines (e.g. interleukins) are endogenous ligands, and Toll-like receptors, for which lipids, lipopeptides, peptidoglycans, and viruses may act as endogenous ligands.

Neurotransmitter systems

Important neurotransmitter systems of the central nervous system are considered briefly in this section.

Dopamine

The primary biosynthetic pathway for dopamine is as follows:

> tyrosine, acted upon by tyrosine hydroxylase →
> 3,4-dihydroxyphenylalanine (DOPA), acted upon by aromatic amino acid decarboxylase (also known as DOPA decarboxylase) →
> dopamine.

An important catabolic pathway begins with the action of the enzyme catechol-O-methyltransferase (COMT):

> dopamine, acted upon by COMT →
> 3-methoxytyramine, acted upon by monoamine oxidase (MAO) →
> homovanillic acid (HVA).

Another important catabolic pathway begins with the action of the enzyme MAO:

> dopamine, acted upon by MAO →
> 3,4-dihydroxyphenylacetaldehyde, acted upon by aldehyde dehydrogenase →
> dihydroxyphenylacetic acid (DOPAC), acted upon by COMT →
> HVA.

Major dopaminergic pathways of the central nervous system include:

- Mesocortical pathway from the ventral tegmental area to the nucleus accumbens and to the cerebral cortex.
- Mesolimbic pathway from the ventral tegmental area to the limbic system.
- Nigrostriatal pathway from the substantia nigra to the caudate nucleus and putamen (that is, to the striatum).
- Tuberinfundibular pathway from the hypothalamic arcuate nucleus and periventricular nucleus to the pituitary gland.

Noradrenaline

The primary biosynthetic pathway for noradrenaline (norepinephrine) is as follows:

> tyrosine, acted upon by tyrosine hydroxylase →
> DOPA, acted upon by aromatic amino acid decarboxylase (DOPA decarboxylase) →
> dopamine, acted upon by dopamine-β-hydroxylase →
> noradrenaline.

An important catabolic pathway begins with the action of COMT:

> noradrenaline, acted upon by COMT →
> normetanephrine, acted upon by MAO →
> 3-methoxy-4-hydroxyphenylglycoaldehyde, acted upon by aldehyde dehydrogenase →
> vanillyl mandelic acid (VMA), which is 3-methoxy-4-hydroxymandelic acid.

Another important catabolic pathway begins with the action of MAO. There are 2 main branches, the first of which is:

> noradrenaline, acted upon by MAO →
> 3,4-dihydroxyphenylglycoaldehyde, acted upon by aldehyde dehydrogenase →
> 3,4-dihydroxymandelic acid, acted upon by COMT →
> VMA.

The second main branch of the catabolic pathway which begins with the action of MAO is:

> noradrenaline, acted upon by MAO →
> 3,4-dihydroxyphenylglycoaldehyde, acted upon by aldehyde reductase →
> 3,4-dihydroxyphenylglycol, acted upon by COMT →
> 3-methoxy-4-hydroxyphenylglycol (MHPG).

Major noradrenergic pathways of the central nervous system include:
- From the locus coeruleus (in the pons): ascending pathways to the hypothalamus, thalamus, olfactory bulb, and cerebral cortex; and descending pathways to the cerebellum and spinal cord.
- From the lateral tegmental nuclei (in the mesencephalon): ascending pathways to the limbic system; and descending pathways to the cerebellum and spinal cord.

Serotonin

The primary biosynthetic pathway for serotonin is as follows:

> tryptophan, acted upon by tryptophan hydroxylase →
> serotonin.

The catabolic pathway of serotonin is:

> serotonin, acted upon by MAO type A (MAOA) →
> 5-hydroxyindoleacetic acid (5-HIAA).

Major serotonergic pathways of the central nervous system include:
- Ascending pathways from the rostral raphe nuclei to the thalamus, limbic system, striatum, and cerebral cortex.
- Descending pathways from the caudal raphe nuclei to the spinal cord.

GABA

The primary biosynthetic pathway for GABA is as follows:

> glutamic acid, acted upon by glutamic acid decarboxylase (GAD) →
> GABA.

The catabolic pathway of GABA is via GABA transaminase (GABA-T) to glutamic acid and succinic semialdehyde.

GABA is usually inhibitory and GABAergic neurons occur widely in the brain.

Glutamate

Glutamate acts as an amino acid neurotransmitter. Glutamate is usually excitatory and glutamergic neurons occur widely in the brain.

Acetylcholine

The biosynthetic pathway for acetylcholine (ACh) is as follows:

$$acetyl\ CoA + choline \rightarrow ACh.$$

This reaction is catalyzed by choline acetyltransferase.

The catabolic pathway of ACh is by hydrolysis, via cholinesterase, resulting in ethanoic acid (also known as acetic acid) + choline.

Major cholinergic pathways of the central nervous system include:

- Ascending pathways from the medial septal nucleus and the nucleus of the diagonal band (in the ventral forebrain) to the hippocampus.
- Ascending pathways from the nucleus basalis (in the ventral forebrain) to the cerebral cortex.
- From brainstem nuclei (in the pons) to the basal forebrain, thalamus, cerebellum, vestibular nuclei, and reticular formation and also to cranial nerve nuclei.
- Striatal interneurons.

Non-depot antipsychotic drugs

Use of antipsychotic drugs 38
Classification of first-generation antipsychotic drugs 40
Second-generation antipsychotic drugs 42
NICE guidance 43
CATIE and CUtLASS 44
Equivalent doses 45
High doses 46
Overall cautions and contraindications 48
Withdrawal of antipsychotic drugs 50
Extrapyramidal symptoms 52
Neuroleptic malignant syndrome 54
Effects of antipsychotic drugs on brain structure 56
Elderly patients 58
Chlorpromazine 60
Trifluoperazine 62
Haloperidol 63
Pimozide 64
Flupentixol 66
Zuclopenthixol 68
Sulpiride 70
Second-generation antipsychotic drugs: side-effects and
     cautions 71
Amisulpride 72
Aripiprazole 74
Clozapine 76
Olanzapine 80
Paliperidone 84
Quetiapine 86
Risperidone 90
Asenapine 93

Use of antipsychotic drugs

Antipsychotic drugs (also known as 'neuroleptics') have a wide variety of uses in psychiatric practice. The main uses of antipsychotic drugs include the treatment of:

- schizophrenia
- bipolar mood disorder—including the acute treatment of mania, hypomania and depression
- severe depression with psychotic features
- psychosis associated with delirium, dementia, or other organic disorders
- psychosis caused by other drugs and by psychoactive substance abuse
- delusional disorders
- symptomatic treatment in disorders such as Huntington's disease
- in the short-term management of violent behaviour.

There are also several non-psychotic uses for antipsychotic drugs, which should be borne in mind when seeing patients. For example, in dermatological practice, 'off-label' prescribing of antipsychotic drugs sometimes occurs for conditions such as pruritus, neurotic excoriations and pathological skin picking, trichotillomania, and cutaneous pain syndromes (including postherpetic neuralgia) (Koo & Ng, 2002).

Classification of first-generation antipsychotic drugs

In general, the older, first-generation, or typical, antipsychotic drugs exhibit antagonistic activity at brain dopaminergic D2 receptors. The main groups are as follows.

Phenothiazines

Phenothiazines have a central tricyclic structure made up of 2 benzene rings covalently bounded to each other through 1 sulphur- and 1 nitrogen-bridge, as shown in Fig. 3.1.

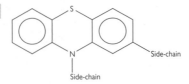

Fig. 3.1 The structure of a phenothiazine.

There are 3 main groups of phenothiazine antipsychotic drugs:
- Those with aliphatic side-chain attached to the nitrogen-bridge, e.g. chlorpromazine, levomepromazine, and promazine. The antipsychotic drugs in this subgroup tend to have a relatively low potency (though they are certainly clinically effective).
- Those with a piperidine ring in the side-chain attached to the phenothiazine nitrogen-bridge, e.g. pipotiazine and pericyazine. These antipsychotic drugs tend to have a depressant action on cardiac conduction and repolarization.
- Those with a piperazine group attached to the nitrogen-bridge, e.g. fluphenazine, trifluoperazine, perphenazine and prochlorperazine.

Table 3.1 shows the general degree of sedative actions and antimuscarinic and extrapyramidal side-effects of these 3 subgroups. The remaining groups of first-generation antipsychotic drugs are listed here tend to resemble phenothiazines with piperazine side-chains in these respects.

Thioxanthenes

Like phenothiazines, thioxanthenes are also tricyclic antipsychotic drugs. The core tricyclic structure is similar to that of the phenothiazines, but with a carbon-bridge rather than a nitrogen-bridge, as shown in Fig. 3.2. Again, two side-chains are attached to this tricyclic structure.

Examples of thioxanthenes include flupentixol and zuclopenthixol, which are both available as depot preparations.

Table 3.1 The general degree of sedative actions and antimuscarinic and extrapyramidal side-effects of the 3 subgroups of phenothiazines

Subgroup	Sedation	Antimuscarinic effects	Extrapyramidal side-effects
Aliphatic	+++	++	++
Piperidine	++	+++	+
Piperazine	+	+	+++

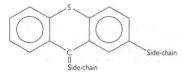

Fig. 3.2 The structure of a thioxanthene.

Butyrophenones

The butyrophenones are phenylbutylpiperidines and include haloperidol and benperidol.

Diphenylbutylpiperidines

The main diphenylbutylpiperidine in clinical psychiatric use in the UK at the time of writing is pimozide. (Others include fluspirilene and penfluridol.)

Substituted benzamides

The main substituted benzamide used as an antipsychotic drug in the UK and many other countries is sulpiride. Some authorities class sulpiride as an atypical antipsychotic drug. Other substituted benzamides include metoclopramide, which is used as an antiemetic drug and which may cause extrapyramidal side-effects, hyperprolactinaemia, tardive dyskinesia, and other side-effects associated with the use of typical antipsychotic drugs. A molecular variant of sulpiride, amisulpride, is also used as an antipsychotic drug, and is a second-generation (or atypical) antipsychotic which is considered in the next section.

Second-generation antipsychotic drugs

In general, the newer, second-generation, or atypical, antipsychotic drugs are associated with less frequent extrapyramidal side-effects than the first-generation antipsychotics. The second-generation antipsychotic drugs currently in routine use in the UK are:

- amisulpride
- aripiprazole
- clozapine
- olanzapine
- paliperidone
- quetiapine
- risperidone.

Clozapine is a dibenzodiazepine and is the archetypal atypical antipsychotic; olanzapine and quetiapine have similar molecular structures. Aripiprazole is a quinolinone derivative while risperidone is a benzisoxazole and paliperidone is an active metabolite of risperidone (paliperidone is 9-hydroxyrisperidone).

NICE guidance

In 2009, the National Institute for Health and Clinical Excellence, known as NICE, which is an independent UK organization responsible for providing national guidance on the promotion of good health and the prevention and treatment of ill health, issued the following guidance on pharmacological interventions for patients suffering from schizophrenia.

'For people with newly diagnosed schizophrenia, offer oral antipsychotic medication. Provide information and discuss the benefits and side-effect profile of each drug with the service user. The choice of drug should be made by the service user and healthcare professional together, considering:
- the relative potential of individual antipsychotic drugs to cause extrapyramidal side effects (including akathisia), metabolic side effects (including weight gain) and other side effects (including unpleasant subjective experiences)
- the views of the carer if the service user agrees.'

Before starting antipsychotic medication, NICE recommend that an electrocardiogram should be carried out if any of the following criteria is met:
- This investigation is specified in the manufacturer's summary of product characteristics.
- A physical examination has identified specific cardiovascular risk (such as hypertension).
- There is a personal history of cardiovascular disease.
- The patient is being admitted as an inpatient.

CATIE and CUtLASS

CATIE and CUtLASS refer to two large studies comparing first-generation antipsychotics with second-generation antipsychotics; both studies were funded independently of pharmaceutical companies.

CATIE (Clinical Antipsychotic Trials of Intervention Effectiveness) was funded by the National Institute of Mental Health (NIMH) and compared the second-generation antipsychotics olanzapine, quetiapine, risperidone and ziprasidone (included in the study after its approval by the US Food and Drug Administration) and the first-generation antipsychotic per-phenazine. Almost 1500 patients with chronic schizophrenia were ran-domly assigned to treatment with one of these antipsychotic drugs in a double-blind design, with the primary outcome measure being discontinu-ation of treatment for any cause (Lieberman et al., 2005). The surprising conclusions of this study were as follows: 'The majority of patients in each group discontinued their assigned treatment owing to inefficacy or intoler-able side effects or for other reasons. Olanzapine was the most effective in terms of the rates of discontinuation, and the efficacy of the conventional antipsychotic agent perphenazine appeared similar to that of quetiapine, risperidone, and ziprasidone. Olanzapine was associated with greater weight gain and increases in measures of glucose and lipid metabolism.'

CUtLASS (Cost Utility of the Latest Antipsychotic drugs in Schizophrenia Study) was funded by the Health Technology Assessment Programme and compared first-generation antipsychotics and second-generation antipsy-chotics (apart from clozapine). 227 patients with schizophrenia and related disorders were assessed for medication review because of inadequate response or adverse effects; the patients were randomly prescribed either first-generation antipsychotics or second-generation antipsychotics (other than clozapine), with the individual medication choice in each arm being made by the patients' psychiatrists (Jones et al., 2006). The study found that patients in the first-generation antipsychotic arm showed a trend toward greater improvement in Quality of Life Scale and symptom scores, and overall patients reported no clear preference for either group of antipsychotics. The authors concluded that: 'In people with schizophrenia whose medication is changed for clinical reasons, there is no disadvantage across 1 year in terms of quality of life, symptoms, or associated costs of care in using [first-generation antipsychotics] rather than nonclozapine [second-generation antipsychotics]. Neither inadequate power nor pat-terns of drug discontinuation accounted for the result.'

Owens (2011) has recently commented as follows on the implications of these two major studies:

'Antipsychotic choices should be based on an 'individual risk:benefit appraisal', where the particular illness, then the individual patient and finally individual drug variables are considered in turn for treatment that is truly 'tailored'. Now, the entire repertoire of antipsychotics can be opened up to equal consideration.

Alas, a whole generation has matured through the specialist ranks with little or no exposure to older antipsychotics. For them, Stelazine [triflu-operazine] might as well be a fizzy drink! A major educational undertaking is necessary.'

Equivalent doses

Equivalent doses for a selection of orally administered antipsychotic drugs are given in the *British National Formulary*, 62nd edition, and reproduced in Table 3.2. They are intended only as an approximate guide. Note that these equivalent doses should not be extrapolated beyond the maximum dose for each antipsychotic drug.

Table 3.2 Equivalent doses of oral antipsychotics. Reproduced with permission from the *British National Formulary*, 62nd edn. BMJ Group & Pharmaceutical Press, London

Antipsychotic	Daily dose
Chlorpromazine	100mg
Clozapine	50mg
Haloperidol	2–3mg
Pimozide	2mg
Risperidone	0.5–1mg
Sulpiride	200mg
Trifluoperazine	5mg

High doses

In the UK, antipsychotic doses which exceed those given in the latest *British National Formulary* are unlicensed. The Royal College of Psychiatrists have issued the following advice on doses exceeding the *British National Formulary* upper limits.

1. Consider alternative approaches including adjuvant therapy and newer or second-generation antipsychotics such as clozapine.
2. Bear in mind risk factors, including obesity; particular caution is indicated in older patients, especially those over 70.
3. Consider potential for drug interactions.
4. Carry out ECG to exclude untoward abnormalities such as prolonged QT interval; repeat ECG periodically and reduce dose if prolonged QT interval or other adverse abnormality develops.
5. Increase dose slowly and not more often than once weekly.
6. Carry out regular pulse, blood pressure, and temperature checks; ensure that patient maintains adequate fluid intake.
7. Consider high-dose therapy to be for limited period and review regularly; abandon if no improvement after 3 months (return to standard dosage).

In addition, the *British National Formulary* offers the following advice:

'**Important:** When prescribing an antipsychotic for administration on an emergency basis, the intramuscular dose should be **lower** than the corresponding oral dose (owing to absence of first-pass effect), particularly if the patient is very active (increased blood flow to muscle considerably increases the rate of absorption). The prescription should specify the dose for **each route** and should **not** imply that the same dose can be given by mouth or by intramuscular injection. The dose of antipsychotic for emergency use should be reviewed at least **daily**.'

Overall cautions and contraindications

Caution

Caution should be exercised when considering prescribing antipsychotic drugs to patients suffering from:
- A propensity to angle-closure glaucoma (including a family history).
- Blood dyscrasias—an urgent blood count should be carried out if a patient being treated with an antipsychotic drug develops an unexplained infection, pyrexia, or malaise; blood dyscrasias can be of rapid onset.
- Cardiovascular disease—many antipsychotic drugs affect the heart (and may prolong the cardiac rate-corrected QT interval, QTc) and blood vasculature directly, while some, such as chlorpromazine, olanzapine and risperidone, can induce orthostatic hypotension.
- Depression.
- Epilepsy (including disorders predisposing to epilepsy)—the seizure threshold is lowered by many antipsychotic drugs and electroencephalographic discharge patterns may occur. It is best not to use antipsychotic drugs, if at all possible, in patients who are withdrawing from alcohol or other drugs that cause central nervous system depression, such as barbiturates and benzodiazepines.
- Jaundice (including a history of this)—jaundice (usually without pruritus) may particularly occur with chlorpromazine treatment.
- Myasthenia gravis.
- Old age—the elderly are particularly susceptible to postural hypotension. Many antipsychotic drugs have a poikilothermic effect, which is probably mediated by hypothalamic actions, such that shivering is inhibited, so reducing the ability of the body to warm up in the cold. The elderly may suffer from hypothermia when it is cold and from hyperthermia when it is very warm.
- Parkinson's disease—many antipsychotic drugs act as dopaminergic antagonists and such action in the basal ganglia can exacerbate pre-existing Parkinson's disease, as well as inducing extrapyramidal effects in patients who do not suffer from this disease.
- Prostatic hypertrophy—in men with this condition, antipsychotic drugs may cause acute urinary retention.
- Renal impairment.
- Respiratory disease, severe. (Note that if a patient—with or without a history of respiratory disease—appears suddenly to have developed an apparent respiratory infection, the possibility of the development of a blood dyscrasia should be considered and an urgent blood count carried out, as mentioned earlier in this list.)

Activities to avoid

The following should be avoided if at all possible:
- Breastfeeding—mothers should not breastfeed while taking antipsychotic drugs as the latter tend to be present in the milk.
- Driving—antipsychotic treatment may be associated with drowsiness, which can clearly be dangerous during driving. Note that antipsychotics can also increase the effects of alcohol.

- Exposure to ultraviolet light—many antipsychotic drugs may cause photosensitization, so that exposure to sunlight and other sources of ultraviolet light (such as sun tanning equipment) should be avoided. Patients who are going to be exposed to direct sunlight should be offered sunscreen creams that block ultraviolet light.
- Operating machinery—see 'Driving', p.48.

Contraindications

Contraindications to the use of antipsychotic drugs include:
- central nervous system depression.
- comatose states.
- phaeochromocytoma.
- pregnancy—unless absolutely necessary.

Withdrawal of antipsychotic drugs

Following long-term antipsychotic drug pharmacotherapy, withdrawal of the drug should take place gradually and under close medical supervision. It is particularly important to look out for evidence of withdrawal syndromes or relapse of the psychiatric illness (for up to 2 years following antipsychotic withdrawal).

Extrapyramidal symptoms

These are particularly likely to occur with the first-generation antipsychotic drugs haloperidol, benperidol, fluphenazine, perphenazine, trifluoperazine, prochlorperazine and first-generation antipsychotic depot medication. The most important extrapyramidal symptoms are:

- acute dystonic reactions
- akathisia
- parkinsonism
- tardive dyskinesia.

In addition, perioral tremor may rarely occur.

Acute dystonic reactions

These can involve abnormal contractions of muscles controlling movements of the tongue, face, mouth, neck and back and of muscles involved in respiratory movements. Clinical manifestations include:

- grimacing
- oculogyric crisis
- opisthotonos
- torticollis
- dystonia of laryngeal and pharyngeal muscles (which may cause death).

In children and adolescents, dyskinesias are commoner than dystonias. Both dystonias and dyskinesias tend to occur acutely, usually after just the initial few doses, within 1–5 days of starting antipsychotic drug pharmacotherapy. They usually respond well to antimuscarinic (anticholinergic or antiparkinsonian) medication, usually parenterally (see Chapter 12).

Acute dystonic reactions may be misdiagnosed as epileptic seizures or even hysteria. The positive response to antimuscarinic medication of acute dystonic reactions may be considered diagnostic.

Akathisia

This is a subjective feeling of motor restlessness, in which the patient experiences a strong urge to move soon after adopting a position associated with being relatively still (such as sitting down, lying down, or adopting a standing position). It tends to occur following large initial antipsychotic drug doses, usually between 5–60 days after starting the treatment. Pharmacological management includes either reducing the antipsychotic dosage or changing antipsychotic drug. Occasionally a beta-blocker or benzodiazepine may need to be used. Note that akathisia is not solely associated with the older typical antipsychotic drugs; atypicals that can cause akathisia include clozapine, risperidone and olanzapine.

Important differential diagnoses are anxiety disorders and agitation. In the case of agitation, it may be appropriate to increase the antipsychotic dose, whereas the dose should be decreased for akathisia.

Parkinsonism

Parkinsonian symptoms may gradually manifest, with the maximum risk being between 5 days and 2 months of starting an antipsychotic drug. They are believed to be caused by antagonism at dopaminergic receptors, particularly in the basal ganglia, and may include:

- bradykinesia
- mask-like facies
- rigidity
- shuffling gait
- tremor
- unsteadiness.

Pharmacological management includes antipsychotic drug dose reduction or withdrawal and antimuscarinic medication (see Chapter 12).

Tardive dyskinesia

In tardive dyskinesia, involuntary abnormal waking (daytime) oro-facio-lin-gual movements which tend to be stereotyped, rhythmic, choreiform, and painless occur, and there may also be more widespread choreoathetoid movements or sustained dystonias. The dyskinesias are usually not present during sleep. Tardive dyskinesia usually occurs after long-term treatment or the use of high doses of antipsychotic drugs, but there have been cases following short-term treatment with low doses of these drugs. The cause is not known, and there is no effective management at present; antipsychotic drug withdrawal may not be effective. The *British National Formulary* makes the following important points:

'…some manufacturers suggest that drug withdrawal at the earliest signs of tardive dyskinesia (fine vermicular movements of the tongue) may halt its full development. Tardive dyskinesia occurs fairly frequently, especially in the elderly, and [antipsychotic drug] treatment must be carefully and regularly reviewed.'

Perioral tremor

Perioral tremor, or rabbit syndrome, is an antipsychotic-induced rhythmic motion of the perioral region (mouth and lips) which is said to resemble the chewing movements of a rabbit. It is relatively rare (occurring in about 2–4% of patients treated with typical antipsychotic drugs) and tends to manifest after months or years of treatment. Its cause is not known. Pharmacological management includes a reduction in antipsychotic drug dosage (as much as is clinically prudent) and, if this is not effective (or not clinically feasible), antimuscarinic medication.

Neuroleptic malignant syndrome

This is a medical emergency that is life-threatening and requires immediate treatment.

Clinical features

The clinical features of neuroleptic malignant syndrome include:
- autonomic dysfunction:
  - hyperthermia
  - labile blood pressure
  - pallor
  - sweating
  - tachycardia
- fluctuating level of consciousness (stupor)
- muscular rigidity
- urinary incontinence.

It may last for up to a week after cessation of the offending antipsychotic drug; in the case of depot antipsychotic medication the neuroleptic malignant syndrome may last longer than a week.

Investigations

Blood tests may show:
- raised serum creatine kinase
- leucocytosis.

Management

This is a clinical emergency. The causative antipsychotic drug should be immediately stopped. The patient should be admitted as an inpatient to a medical ward where maximal supportive care should be instituted. Sometimes dantrolene or bromocriptine (a dopamine agonist) may be required.

Prognosis

There may be complications such as renal failure or respiratory failure. The overall mortality is greater than 10%.

Effects of antipsychotic drugs on brain structure

David Lewis' group have found that chronic exposure (over 17–27 months) of macaque monkeys to the orally administered antipsychotic drugs haloperidol or olanzapine, with plasma antipsychotic levels comparable to those achieved in human patients treated with these drugs for schizophrenia, is associated with reduced brain volume (Dorph-Petersen et al., 2005), compared with a third group which received sham treatment. This group also reported a statistically significant 21% lower astrocyte number and a non-significant 13% lower oligodendrocyte number in the grey matter in the antipsychotic-exposed monkeys (the haloperidol and olanzapine groups were similar) (Konopaske et al., 2008). It is noteworthy that these findings are consistent with reports from some post-mortem studies in schizophrenia (Puri, 2011).

From the large cohort of schizophrenia patients who have undergone longitudinal MRI examinations in the Iowa Longitudinal Study, significant progressive brain changes, associated with antipsychotic use, were found in most brain regions (Ho et al., 2011). These have been summarized by Puri (2011):

'[These changes included] reductions in volume in: total cerebral tissue; total cerebral grey matter; frontal grey matter; temporal grey matter; parietal grey matter; caudate; putamen; and thalamus. Significant increases in volume were found in: parietal white matter; lateral ventricles; and sulcal cerebrospinal fluid (CSF). After adjusting for the potential confounding effects of the other three predictor variables [follow-up duration, illness severity and alcohol or illicit drug misuse], antipsychotic treatment was found to have significant main effects on total cerebral and lobar grey matter and putamen volumes; higher antipsychotic medication dose was associated with smaller total cerebral, frontal, temporal, and parietal grey matter volumes (all independent of follow-up duration), and with a larger putamen volume. Significant treatment × time interaction effects were found for total cerebral tissue volumes, total cerebral and lobar white matter, lateral ventricular, sulcal CSF, caudate, putamen, and cerebellar volumes. Greater antipsychotic dose was associated with greater reduction in white matter, caudate, and cerebellar volumes over time, and with greater CSF volume and putamen enlargement. There were no significant main effects of the severity of alcohol or illicit substance misuse on brain volume changes apart from the lateral ventricles (increased in size) and the cerebellar volumes (decreased).'

The group also examined the issue of whether any particular type of antipsychotic drug was particularly associated with changes in brain structure (or, indeed, a lack of such an association). They split the antipsychotic drugs into the following three groups: first-generation antipsychotics, clozapine, and non-clozapine second-generation antipsychotics (Ho et al. 2011). These results have been summarized by Puri (2011):

'All three classes of drug were found to be associated with significant changes in brain volumes. Higher typical antipsychotic doses were associated with smaller total cerebral grey matter and frontal grey matter volumes and with higher putamen volumes; higher doses of non-clozapine atypical antipsychotics were associated with lower frontal and parietal grey matter volumes and with higher parietal white matter, caudate, and putamen volumes; higher clozapine doses were associated with smaller total cerebral and lobar grey matter volumes and with larger sulcal CSF volumes and smaller caudate, putamen, and thalamic volumes.'

Elderly patients

The *British National Formulary* points out that antipsychotics are associated, in elderly patients with dementia, with 'a small increased risk of mortality and an increased risk of stroke or transient ischaemic attack.' It also points out that elderly patients have a particular susceptibility to:
- postural hypotension
- hyperthermia
- hypothermia.

The *British National Formulary* recommends the following in respect of antipsychotic medication in elderly patients.
- Such medication should not be used to treat mild to moderate psychotic symptomatology.
- Initial doses should be reduced (≤ half the adult dose) and factor in body mass, comorbidity, and any other medication being taken.
- It should be regularly reviewed.

Chlorpromazine

༄ Structure

Chlorpromazine is the archetypal typical antipsychotic. It is a pheno-thiazine with an aliphatic side-chain attached to the nitrogen-bridge. Its molecular structure is shown in Fig. 3.3.

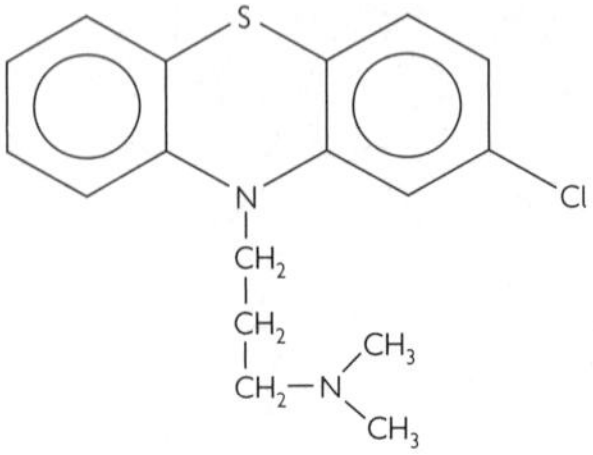

Fig. 3.3 The structure of chlorpromazine hydrochloride.

♪ Dose

The adult oral antipsychotic dose is usually between 75–300mg daily. Up to 1000mg (1g) may be required daily in extreme cases. The doses used in the elderly are a third to a half of these doses.

For children aged between 1–6 years, the recommended *British National Formulary* dose is 500 micrograms per kilogram body mass every 4–6 hours, up to a maximum of 40mg daily. For children aged between 6–12 years, the maximum dose recommended is 75mg daily.

The antipsychotic dose by deep intramuscular injection for adults is 25–50mg every 6–8 hours. For children, the recommended *British National Formulary* dose is 500 micrograms per kilogram body mass every 6–8 hours, up to a maximum of 40mg daily for those aged between 1–6 years, and up to a maximum of 75mg daily for those aged between 6–12 years.

For rectal administration, 100mg chlorpromazine base in the form of a rectal suppository should be taken to be the equivalent of 20–25mg chlorpromazine hydrochloride by intramuscular injection, and the equivalent of 40–50mg chlorpromazine base or chlorpromazine hydrochloride orally.

☺ Side-effects

Chlorpromazine has a wide range of side-effects, many of which are thought to relate to antagonist activity to neurotransmission by:
• dopamine
• acetylcholine—muscarinic receptors
• adrenaline/noradrenaline
• histamine.

Antidopaminergic action on the tuberoinfundibular pathway (see Chapter 2) can lead to hyperprolactinaemia owing to the prolactin-inhibitory factor action of dopamine. In turn, hyperprolactinaemia can lead to:

- galactorrhoea
- gynaecomastia
- menstrual disturbances
- reduced sperm count
- reduced libido.

Antidopaminergic action on the nigrostriatal pathway (see Chapter 2), which has important functions relating to sensorimotor coordination, can cause extrapyramidal symptoms. These have been described earlier.

Central antimuscarinic (anticholinergic) actions may give rise to:

- convulsions
- pyrexia.

Peripheral antimuscarinic (anticholinergic) actions may cause:

- blurred vision
- dry mouth
- constipation
- nasal congestion
- urinary retention.

Antiadrenergic actions can lead to:

- ejaculatory failure
- postural hypotension.

Antihistaminic actions can cause sedation and drowsiness.

Other side-effects of chlorpromazine include:

- allergic (sensitivity) reactions
- blood dyscrasias such as agranulocytosis and leucopenia
- cardiovascular symptoms, such as hypotension, tachycardia, and arrhythmias
- electrocardiographic changes
- gastrointestinal disturbance
- headache
- hypothermia or pyrexia
- jaundice
- photosensitization
- weight gain
- the effects of long-term high-dose treatment, including opacity of the ocular lens and/or cornea and a purplish pigmentation of the skin, conjunctiva, cornea, and retina.

Trifluoperazine

✿ Structure

Trifluoperazine is a phenothiazine with a piperazine group attached to the nitrogen-bridge. Its molecular structure is shown in Fig. 3.4.

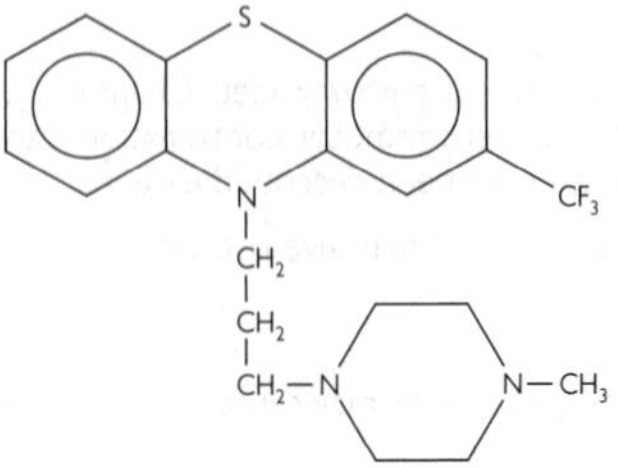

Fig. 3.4 The structure of trifluoperazine.

♪ Dose

The adult oral antipsychotic dose is initially 10mg daily (as 5mg twice daily). Depending on the clinical response, the dose may be increased by 5mg daily after 1 week, and then by another 5mg after a further 3 days. The doses used in the elderly are reduced by a factor of at least one-half of these doses.

☺ Side-effects

As given earlier in the chapter. Compared with chlorpromazine, trifluoperazine is far less sedating and far less likely to cause hypotension, but more likely to cause extrapyramidal symptoms (especially when the daily dose is greater than 6mg).

Trifluoperazine is also particularly associated with:
- anorexia
- hyperpyrexia
- pancytopenia
- thrombocytopenia.

Haloperidol

ஃ Structure

Haloperidol is a butyrophenone. Its molecular structure is shown in Fig. 3.5.

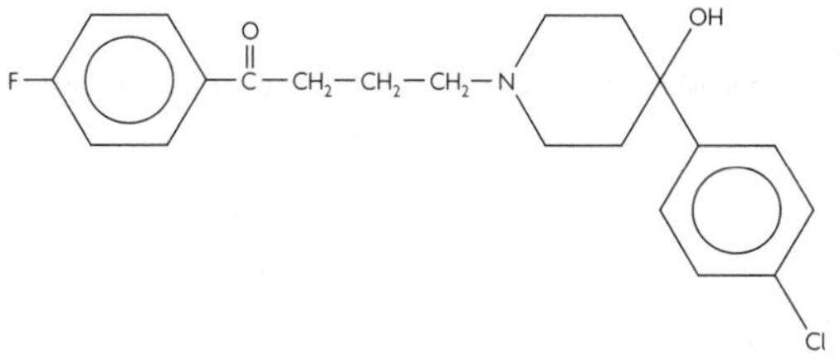

Fig. 3.5 The structure of haloperidol.

Dose

The adult oral antipsychotic dose is initially between 0.5–3mg twice or thrice daily, making a maximum total of 9mg daily. In severe or resistant cases the initial dose may be as high as 5mg thrice daily, making a maximum total of 15mg per day. (Up to 30mg may initially be required daily in extreme cases of resistant schizophrenia.) The doses used in the elderly are a half of these doses.

For children from the age of 5 years upwards (e.g. for Tourette syndrome), the initial oral dose is 25–50 micrograms per kilogram body mass daily, up to a maximum of 10mg daily.

The antipsychotic dose by intramuscular or intravenous injection for adults is initially 2–10mg, and then every 4–8 hours, depending on the clinical response, up to a maximum of 18mg daily in total. Again, the doses used in the elderly are a half of these doses. Intramuscular and intravenous injection of haloperidol are not recommended for children.

Side-effects

As given earlier in the chapter. Compared with chlorpromazine, haloperidol is far less sedating, far less likely to cause hypotension, and less likely to cause antimuscarinic symptoms, but more likely to cause extrapyramidal symptoms.

Haloperidol has been reported to be associated with:

- hypoglycaemia
- inappropriate antidiuretic hormone secretion
- weight loss.

Pimozide

Pimozide is rarely used as a first-line treatment for schizophrenia. Its use has been associated with sudden death, as described in 'Side effects'. However, it does have a place in the pharmacotherapy of monosymptomatic hypochondriacal psychosis.

⚭ Structure

Pimozide is a diphenylbutylpiperidine. Its molecular structure is shown in Fig. 3.6.

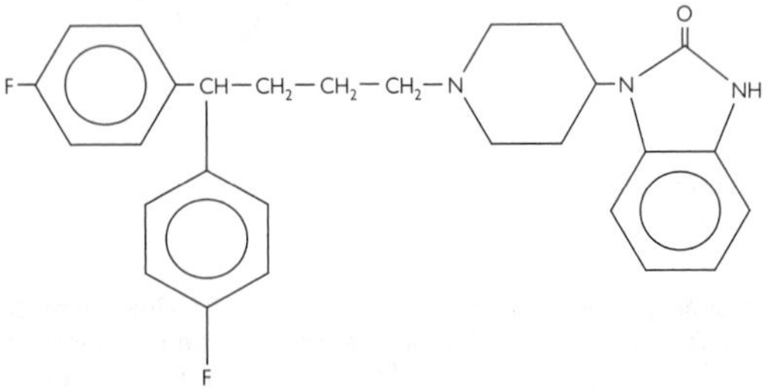

Fig. 3.6 The structure of pimozide.

♣ Dose

For schizophrenia the initial oral daily dose is 2mg. This can be increased, no more quickly than weekly, by 2–4mg per day to a maximum of 20mg daily. For monosymptomatic hypochondriacal psychosis and paranoid psychosis, the initial daily dose is 4mg, which can be increased, no more quickly than weekly, by 2–4mg per day to a maximum of 16mg daily.

For the elderly, half these initial starting doses are used, that is, 1mg daily for schizophrenia and 2mg daily for monosymptomatic hypochondriacal psychosis and paranoid psychosis.

Pimozide is not recommended for use in children.

☹ Side-effects

As given earlier in the chapter. Compared with chlorpromazine, pimozide is far less sedating and far less likely to cause hypotension, but more likely to cause extrapyramidal symptoms.

Treatment with pimozide has been reported to be associated with sudden unexplained death. In the UK, the CSM have recommended that:
- An ECG be carried out before starting treatment with pimozide.
- An annual ECG be carried out while on treatment with pimozide.
- If there is QT interval prolongation the pimozide should be withdrawn or its dose reduced under close supervision.
- Pimozide should not be prescribed with:
  - other antipsychotic drugs (including depot injection preparations)
  - tricyclic antidepressants
  - other drugs which prolong the QT interval, such as:

    — certain antimalarials
    — antiarrhythmic drugs
    — certain antihistamines
- drugs which cause electrolyte disturbances, such as diuretics.

Pimozide has also been reported to be associated with:
- glycosuria
- hyponatraemia.

Flupentixol

In the UK and USA, flupentixol used to be known as flupenthixol.

⚛ Structure

Flupentixol is a thioxanthene. Its molecular structure is shown in Fig. 3.7.

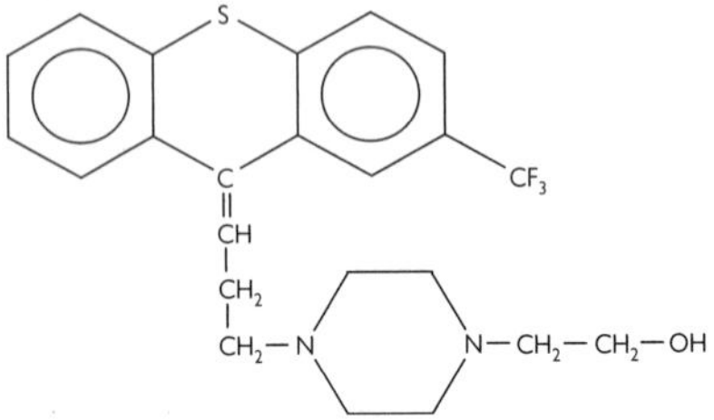

Fig. 3.7 The structure of flupentixol.

⚖ Dose

The adult oral antipsychotic dose is initially between 3–9mg twice daily, making a maximum total of 18mg daily. The doses used in the elderly or debilitated are initially a quarter to a half of these doses.

Flupentixol is not recommended for use in children.

☹ Side-effects

As given earlier in the chapter. Flupentixol is less sedating than chlorpromazine but frequently gives rise to extrapyramidal symptoms.

Zuclopenthixol

In some countries zuclopenthixol is known as clopenthixol.

℘ Structure

Like flupentixol, zuclopenthixol is a thioxanthene. Its molecular structure, shown in Fig. 3.8, is similar to that of flupentixol (see Fig. 3.7, p.66).

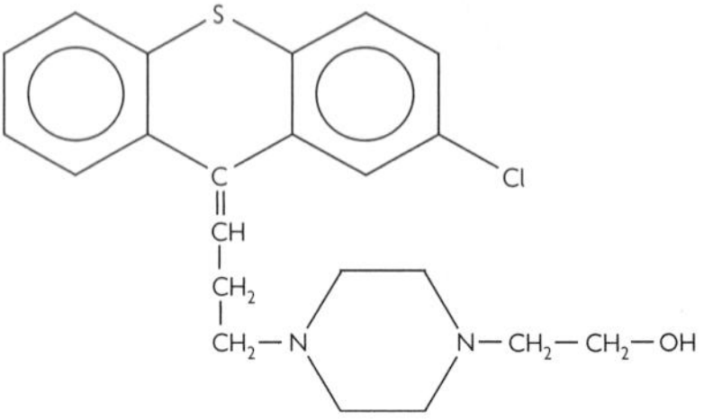

Fig. 3.8 The structure of zuclopenthixol.

♣ Dose

In the UK, zuclopenthixol is available in 3 forms:
- Tablets of zuclopenthixol dihydrochloride for oral use as an antipsychotic drug particularly in cases of agitation, aggression, and hostility.
- An injectable form of zuclopenthixol acetate for deep intramuscular injection in the short-term treatment of acute psychosis, mania or exacerbations of chronic psychosis.
- An injectable depot preparation of zuclopenthixol decanoate, which is described in Chapter 4 (p.109).

The initial adult daily antipsychotic oral dose of zuclopenthixol dihydro-chloride is 20–30mg, administered in divided doses, with a maximum total daily dose of 150mg but a more usual maintenance daily dose of 20–50mg. The doses used in the elderly or debilitated are initially a quarter to a half of these doses.

The initial adult intramuscular dose of zuclopenthixol acetate is 50–150mg. This should be administered by deep intramuscular injection into the upper outer quadrant of the gluteal region (to reduce the risk of damage to the sciatic nerve) or into the lateral thigh. For the elderly, the initial intramuscular dose of zuclopenthixol acetate is 50–100mg. A second intramuscular dose may be required clinically 1–2 days later. The injections may be repeated, if required clinically, every 2–3 days, so long as the maximum total (cumulative) dose given is 400mg in 2 weeks, with a maximum total of 4 injections and a maximum length of treatment-course of 2 weeks. (If maintenance is required clinically on an antipsychotic drug at the end of this course of treatment, then oral zuclopenthixol dihydro-chloride may be given 2–3 days after the last injection of zuclopenthixol acetate, or alternatively a depot antipsychotic drug may be administered with the last injection of zuclopenthixol acetate.)

Zuclopenthixol is not recommended for use in children.

☺ Side-effects

As given earlier in the chapter. Zuclopenthixol should be avoided in patients with porphyria. Orally administered zuclopenthixol dihydrochloride has been associated with:

- urinary frequency or urinary incontinence
- weight loss (although weight gain is a more common side-effect).

Sulpiride

℘ Structure

Sulpiride is a substituted benzamide. Its molecular structure is shown in Fig. 3.9.

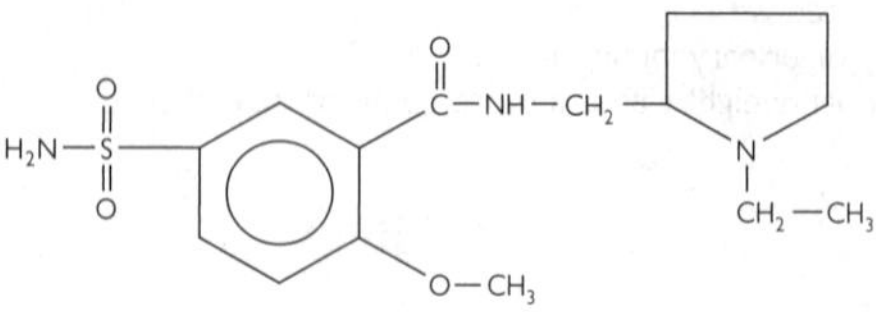

Fig. 3.9 The structure of sulpiride.

♪ Dose

The adult oral antipsychotic dose is usually between 200–400mg twice daily, making a maximum total of 800mg daily (for schizophrenia characterized by mainly negative symptoms). For schizophrenia characterized by mainly positive symptoms, the maximum daily dose can reach 2400mg or 2.4 g. The doses used in the elderly are initially lower, with any increases determined by clinical response.

Sulpiride is not recommended for use in children under the age of 14 years.

☺ Side-effects

As given earlier in the chapter. Sulpiride has been associated with:
• hepatitis.

Second-generation antipsychotic drugs: side-effects and cautions

☺ Side-effects

General side-effects of second-generation antipsychotics include:
- weight gain
- hyperglycaemia—e.g. with clozapine and olanzapine
- type 2 diabetes mellitus can occur—e.g. with clozapine and olanzapine
- dizziness
- postural hypotension (especially during initial dose titration) which may be associated with syncope or reflex tachycardia
- extrapyramidal symptoms (usually mild and transient and which respond to dose reduction or to an antimuscarinic drug) but occasionally tardive dyskinesia following long-term treatment
- neuroleptic malignant syndrome (rare).

Body mass and plasma glucose should be monitored regularly, in view of the risk of hyperglycaemia, metabolic syndrome and type 2 diabetes mellitus.

Cautions

Antipsychotic drugs should be used with caution in patients who:
- have a history of cardiovascular disease
- are being prescribed other drugs which prolong the QT interval, such as:
  - certain antimalarials
  - antiarrhythmic drugs
  - certain antihistamines
- have a history of epilepsy
- are elderly.

Amisulpride

⚥ Structure

Amisulpride is an atypical antipsychotic drug which is a molecular variant of the substituted benzamide sulpride. Its molecular structure is shown in Fig. 3.10.

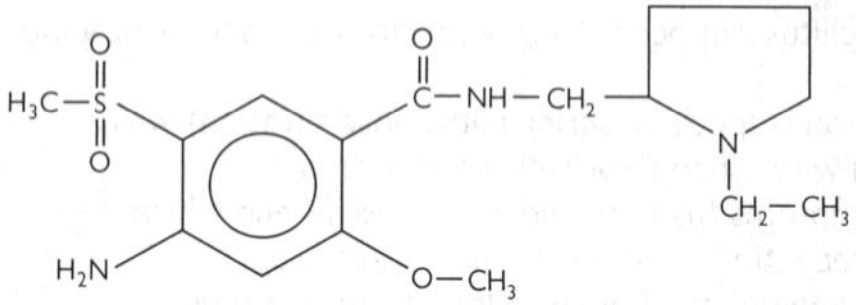

Fig. 3.10 The structure of amisulpride.

⚘ Receptor binding

Amisulpride has a high affinity for:

- dopamine D_2 receptors
- dopamine D_3 receptors.

Amisulpride shows essentially no affinity to other dopaminergic receptors or to central serotonergic, muscarinic cholinergic, histaminergic, or adrenergic receptors. Furthermore, its selective binding to dopamine D_2 and D_3 receptors occurs preferentially in the limbic system (rather than the striatum), thereby possibly accounting for its low propensity to cause extrapyramidal symptoms. While low doses of amisulpride block presynaptic D_2 and D_3 autoreceptors, and so increase dopaminergic neurotransmission, high doses block postsynaptic receptors, and so inhibit dopaminergic hyperactivity.

⚑ Dose

The daily adult oral antipsychotic dose is usually between 400–800mg, in divided doses, with a maximum total of 1200mg or 1.2 g daily, according to clinical response. For schizophrenia characterized by mainly negative symptoms, the daily adult dose is usually between 50–300mg

Amisulpride is not recommended for use in children under the age of 15 years.

☺ Side-effects

As given earlier in the chapter. Amisulpride is also associated with:

- agitation
- anxiety
- bradycardia
- constipation
- drowsiness
- dry mouth
- insomnia.

- nausea
- tic-like symptoms
- vomiting.

Amisulpride may also cause hyperprolactinaemia, which in turn may be associated with:
- amenorrhoea
- breast pain
- galactorrhoea
- gynaecomastia
- sexual dysfunction.

In addition to the cautions given (in respect of second-generation antipsychotic drugs generally), in the case of amisulpride caution should also be exercised in the following cases:
- renal impairment
- Parkinson's disease.

Contraindications include:
- breastfeeding
- phaeochromocytoma
- pregnancy
- prolactin-dependent tumours.

Aripiprazole

✌ Structure

The molecular structure of aripiprazole is shown in Fig. 3.11.

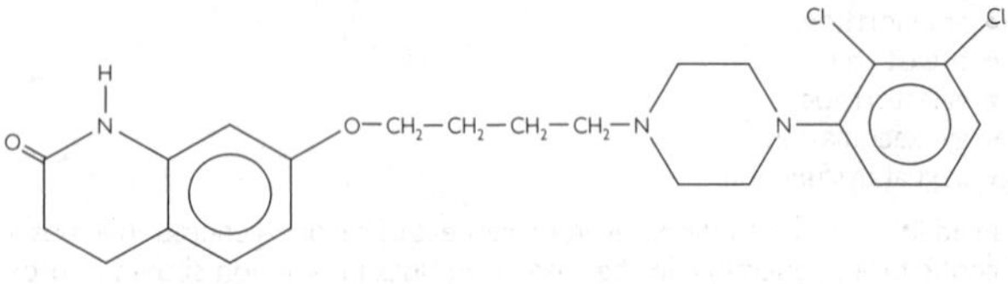

Fig. 3.11 The structure of aripirazole.

⟲ Receptor binding

Aripiprazole has a high affinity for:

- dopamine D_2 receptors—aripiprazole is a partial agonist here
- dopamine D_3 receptors
- serotonin 5-HT_{1A} receptors—aripiprazole is a partial agonist here
- serotonin 5-HT_{1B} receptors.

It has moderate affinity for:

- serotonin 5-HT_{2C} receptors
- serotonin 5-HT_7 receptors
- dopamine D_4 receptors
- α_1-adrenergic receptors
- histamine H_1 receptors
- serotonin reuptake sites.

Aripiprazole is also an antagonist at serotonin 5-$HT2_A$ receptors. It has essentially no affinity for cholinergic muscarinic receptors.

♣ Dose

The daily adult oral antipsychotic dose is 10–15mg, once daily. If the clinical condition requires it, the dose can be increased to a maximum of 30mg once daily.

For children aged between 15–18 years, the initial dose is 2mg once daily for 2 days, followed by 5mg once daily for another 2 days, and then increasing to 10mg daily.

Aripiprazole is not recommended for use in children under the age of 15 years.

☺ Side-effects

The commonest side-effects are:

- insomnia
- headache
- akathisia
- asthenia

- nausea
- vomiting
- dyspepsia
- constipation
- somnolence
- fatigue
- tremor
- blurred vision
- tachycardia.

In addition to the cautions given (in respect of second-generation antipsychotic drugs generally), in the case of aripiprazole caution should also be exercised in the following cases:
- elderly
- hepatic impairment
- cerebrovascular disease
- pregnancy.

Contraindications include:
- breastfeeding.

Clozapine

℣ Structure

Clozapine is the archetypal atypical antipsychotic drug. It is a tricyclic dibenzodiazepine derivative, with the molecular structure shown in Fig. 3.12.

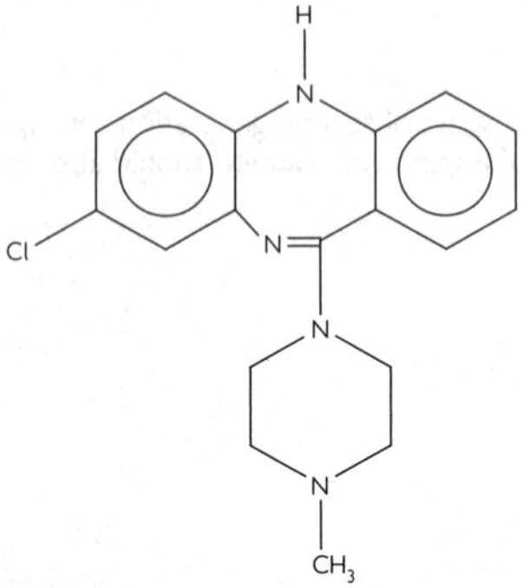

Fig. 3.12 The structure of clozapine.

⊹ Receptor binding

Clozapine has a high affinity for:
- dopamine D_4 receptors
- serotonin $5\text{-}HT_{2A}$ receptors
- serotonin $5\text{-}HT_{2C}$ receptors
- muscarinic cholinergic M_1 receptors
- muscarinic cholinergic M_4 receptors
- α_1-adrenergic receptors
- histamine H_1 receptors.

It has low to moderate affinity for:
- dopamine D_1 receptors
- dopamine D_2 receptors
- dopamine D_3 receptors
- dopamine D_5 receptors
- serotonin $5\text{-}HT_{1A}$ receptors
- serotonin $5\text{-}HT_3$ receptors
- α_2-adrenergic receptors
- muscarinic cholinergic M_2 receptors.

It may have greater activity at limbic rather than striatal dopaminergic receptors, so reducing its extrapyramidal side-effects.

Initiation and blood count monitoring

The daily adult oral antipsychotic dose is usually 200–450mg daily. Initiation of pharmacotherapy with clozapine for the first time must take place under close medical supervision. There is a risk of fatal myocarditis (particularly during the first 2 months) and cardiomyopathy, leading to the following advice from the UK CSM:

- Perform physical examination and take full medical history before starting clozapine.
- Specialist examination if cardiac abnormalities or history of heart disease found—clozapine initiated only in absence of severe heart disease and if benefit outweighs risk.
- Persistent tachycardia especially in first 2 months should prompt observation for other indicators for myocarditis or cardiomyopathy.
- If myocarditis or cardiomyopathy suspected clozapine should be stopped and patient evaluated urgently by a cardiologist.
- Discontinue permanently in clozapine-induced myocarditis or cardiomyopathy.

Since there is also a risk of neutropenia and agranulocytosis (which may be fatal), blood count monitoring is mandatory. It is recommended that the following procedure be carried out in starting an adult (non-elderly) patient on clozapine for the first time:

- Before commencing treatment, check that the leucocyte and differential blood counts are normal. Medical history and full cardiovascular examination.
- Day 1: 12.5mg once or twice daily. Check cardiovascular system (e.g. for hypotension).
- Day 2: 25 to 50mg. Check cardiovascular system.
- Day 3 onwards: gradually increase, if tolerated well, by 25–50mg daily up to 300mg daily (in divided doses, with perhaps a weighting towards the bedtime dose of up to 200mg nocte) over 2–3 weeks. Check cardiovascular system.
- At 1 week: check that the leucocyte and differential blood counts remain normal. Check cardiovascular system.
- At 2 weeks: check that the leucocyte and differential blood counts remain normal. Check cardiovascular system.
- After 2–3 weeks: if clinically necessary, the dose can be increased further, by 50 to 100mg once weekly (or, at most, twice weekly).
- At 3 weeks: check that the leucocyte and differential blood counts remain normal. Check cardiovascular system.
- While the usual daily antipsychotic dose is 200–450mg, the maximum dose is 900mg daily.
- Continue to check that check that the leucocyte and differential blood counts remain normal every week for the first 18 weeks, and then at least once every fortnight until the end of 1 year of treatment. Check cardiovascular system regularly.
- After 1 year: if they remain stable, check the leucocyte and differential blood counts at least once every 4 weeks while on treatment with clozapine. Check cardiovascular system regularly.

For elderly patients, the dose on day 1 should be 12.5mg once. Increases in dosages thereafter should not exceed 25mg per day.

For patients over the age of 16 years who are psychotic and also suffer from Parkinson's disease, the initial dose is 12.5mg nocte. This may be increased by no more than 12.5mg twice weekly to a usual maximum of 50mg nocte, although the usual dose is between 25–37.5mg nocte.

Withdrawal

The blood count should be monitored for 4 weeks following withdrawal of treatment with clozapine, which should take place gradually over 1–2 weeks. (Sudden cessation may be associated with rebound psychosis.)

☺ Side-effects

As given in 'Second-generation antipsychotic drugs: side-effects and cautions', p.71. Also, as mentioned in this section, clozapine may cause the following potentially fatal side-effects:

- agranulocytosis—out-patients should ideally attend a specialized clozapine clinic where their blood counts can be regularly monitored (as indicated earlier) and their cardiovascular system checked. Clozapine treatment should be stopped for good, and a haematology referral made, if the leucocyte count falls below 3000mm^{-3} or the absolute neutrophil count falls below 1500mm^{-3}
- myocarditis and cardiomyopathy.
- seizures.

Other side-effects include:
- agitation
- blurred vision
- cardiac arrest
- cardiac arrhythmia
- circulatory collapse
- convulsions
- delirium
- dermatological reactions
- dizziness
- drowsiness
- dry mouth
- dysphagia
- electrocardiographic changes
- eosinophilia
- extrapyramidal symptoms
- fatigue
- fulminant hepatic necrosis
- gastrointestinal obstruction—patients should be monitored for constipation
- headache
- hepatitis
- hypercholesterolaemia
- hyperglycaemia
- hypersalivation—which may cause dampening of the pillow at night
- hypertension
- hypertriglyceridaemia
- impairment of temperature regulation
- interstitial nephritis
- intestinal obstruction

- jaundice, cholestatic
- leucocytosis
- leucopenia
- nausea
- orthostatic hypotension—with or without syncope
- pancreatitis
- paralytic ileus
- parotid gland enlargement
- pericarditis
- priapism
- pulmonary embolism
- pyrexia
- respiratory arrest
- rigidity
- sweating
- tachycardia
- thrombocythaemia
- thrombocytopenia
- thromboembolism
- tic-like symptoms
- tremor
- urinary incontinence
- urinary retention
- vomiting.

Contraindications include:
- severe cardiac disorders or a history of circulatory collapse—owing to the possibility of myocarditis and cardiomyopathy
- acute hepatic disease
- severe renal impairment
- narrow-angle glaucoma—owing to the anticholinergic actions
- a history of neutropenia, agranulocytosis or bone-marrow disorder
- paralytic ileus—owing to gastrointestinal obstruction; exercise caution if there is a history of colon disease or bowel surgery
- prostate enlargement—owing to the anticholinergic actions
- alcoholic and toxic psychosis and drug intoxication
- central nervous system depression (including coma)
- uncontrolled epilepsy
- pregnancy
- breastfeeding.

Patients taking clozapine should not be given drugs which depress leucopoiesis, and clozapine should be used with caution in patients receiving drugs which cause constipation (including antimuscarinic medication).

Olanzapine

֍ Structure

Olanzapine is a thienobenzodiazepine, with the molecular structure shown in Fig. 3.13.

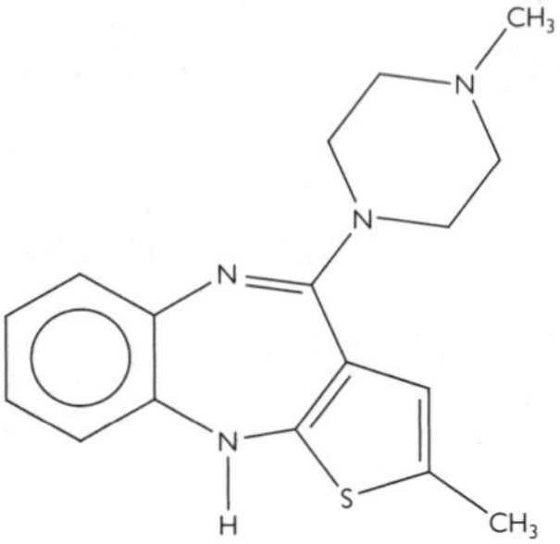

Fig. 3.13 The structure of olanzapine.

֍ Receptor binding

Olanzapine has a high affinity for:
- serotonin 5-HT$_{2A}$ receptors
- serotonin 5-HT$_6$ receptors
- histamine H$_1$ receptors
- serotonin 5-HT$_{2C}$ receptors
- dopamine D$_1$ to D$_4$ receptors
- α_1-adrenergic receptors.

Olanzapine has moderate affinity for:
- muscarinic cholinergic M$_1$ to M$_5$ receptors
- serotonin 5-HT$_3$ receptors.

It has a low affinity for:
- GABA$_A$ receptors
- BZD receptors
- β-adrenergic receptors.

These binding characteristics may help to explain some of the side-effects of olanzapine; for example:
- antimuscarinic (anticholinergic) side-effects—antagonism of M$_1$ to M$_5$ receptors
- somnolence—antagonism of H$_1$ receptors
- orthostatic hypotension—antagonism of α_1-adrenergic receptors.

֍ Dose

The daily adult oral antipsychotic dose is usually between 5–20mg, once daily, based on clinical status. The usual starting oral dose is 10mg once daily, and the maximum is 20mg daily. The drug is often administered in the early evening. For the following patient groups a starting antipsychotic oral dose of 5mg once daily should be considered, and any increase in dose thereafter should be gradual:

- debilitated patients
- predisposition to hypotensive reactions
- pharmacological sensitivity to olanzapine
- female—drug clearance is, on average, around 30% lower than in men
- elderly—the average elimination half-life is around one-and-a-half times greater in those aged over 65 years than in younger adults
- non-smokers—drug clearance is, on average, around 40% higher in smokers than in non-smokers.

In addition to ordinary tablets, oral administration can also be carried out using orodispersible tablets (known as Velotab® in the UK and Zydis® in the USA) which dissolve quickly after being placed on the tongue. They have the following advantages over ordinary tablets:

- Rapidly dissolve in the mouth.
- Do not have to be taken with a drink.
- Can be used in patients who have difficulty in swallowing tablets.
- Improves compliance by reducing the risk of the medication being spat out or being hidden under the tongue or within a cheek.
- Bioequivalent to ordinary olanzapine tablets.
- Can be pre-dissolved in a drink such as water, orange juice, apple juice, milk, or coffee.

Olanzapine is also available in an injectable form for intramuscular administration, for the treatment of agitation and disturbed behaviour in schizophrenia (and also for the treatment of agitation and disturbed behaviour in mania—see Chapter 5). The recommended adult intramuscular dose for agitation in schizophrenia is initially 5–10mg (as one dose), followed by 5–10mg by intramuscular injection after 2 hours if clinically necessary. The total oral and intramuscular dose should not exceed 20mg daily.

For at least 4 hours following intramuscular injection of olanzapine, the following should be monitored:

- pulse
- blood pressure
- respiratory rate.

The recommended initial intramuscular dose is 2.5–5mg in the following groups:

- elderly patients
- debilitated patients
- predisposition to hypotensive reactions
- pharmacological sensitivity to olanzapine
- female—dose reductions are not routinely recommended in women, but the combined effect of being female with one of the other factors listed here may require dose reduction
- non-smokers—dose reductions are not routinely recommended in non-smokers, but the combined effect of being a non-smoker with one of the other factors listed here may warrant dose reduction.

In these groups, a maximum of 3 injections of 2.5 to 5mg daily for 3 days should be given, and a maximum total oral and intramuscular dose of 20mg daily should not be exceeded.

The preparation for intramuscular injection is available in the form of a powder for reconstitution with sterile water into a liquid with a concentration of 5mg olanzapine per 1mL solution. Each vial contains 10mg olanzapine (to be made up to 2mL). The solution should be clear when made up, and should be used within 1 hour of reconstitution.

Laboratory testing

In patients with significant hepatic disease, it is prudent to assess the levels of transaminases regularly.

☹ Side-effects

See the section on side-effects and cautions with antipsychotic drugs, p.71. Also, as mentioned earlier in relation to the receptor binding of olanzapine, it also causes antimuscarinic (anticholinergic) side-effects, somnolence and orthostatic hypotension. Other relatively common side-effects of olanzapine include:

- akathisia
- asthenia
- gait abnormality
- hallucinations
- hyperprolactinaemia
- increased appetite
- increased cough
- peripheral oedema
- pyrexia
- raised triglyceride levels
- speech difficulties
- worsening of Parkinson's disease.

Uncommon side-effects include:
- bradycardia
- hypotension
- photosensitivity
- QT prolongation
- urinary incontinence.

Intramuscular injection may additionally give rise to:
- hypoventilation
- reactions at the injection site
- sinus pause.

In addition to those alreadygiven, caution should also be exercised in the following cases:
- bone-marrow depression
- diabetes mellitus
- hepatic impairment
- hypereosinophilic disorders
- low leucocyte count
- low neutrophil count

- myeloproliferative disease
- paralytic ileus
- Parkinson's disease
- pregnancy
- prostatic hypertrophy
- renal impairment.

Contraindications include:
- angle-closure glaucoma
- breastfeeding.

Contraindications to intramuscular olanzapine injection include:
- acute myocardial infarction
- recent cardiac surgery
- severe bradycardia
- severe hypotension
- sick sinus syndrome
- unstable angina.

Signs of respiratory depression should be monitored following intramuscular injection, including the pulse, respiratory rate and blood pressure, for at least 4 hours following the injection.

Paliperidone

ஃ Structure

Paliperidone is an active metabolite of the benzisoxazole derivative risperidone (see Fig. 3.15, p.90); paliperidone is 9-hydroxyrisperidone.

⊹ Receptor binding

The receptor binding properties of paliperidone are similar to those of risperidone (see p.90).

⌁ Dose

For adults (>18 years), the usual starting dose is 6mg mane, adjusted in steps of 3mg over a period of ≥5 days to a total daily dose of between 3–12mg.

Paliperidone is also available in an injectable depot form, which is described in Chapter 4 (p.106).

☺ Side-effects

See the section on side-effects and cautions with antipsychotic drugs, p.71. Relatively common side-effects of paliperidone include:
- abdominal pain
- agitation
- asthenia
- bradycardia
- bundle branch block
- drowsiness
- dry mouth
- first-degree AV block
- headache
- hypersalivation
- tachycardia
- vomiting.

Less common side-effects include:
- arrhythmias
- erectile dysfunction
- galactorrhoea
- gynaecomastia
- ischaemia
- menstrual disturbances
- nightmares
- oedema
- palpitations
- rash
- seizures
- syncope.

In addition to those given here (including exercising caution in elderly patients who have dementia and have risk factors for developing a stroke), caution should also be exercised in the following cases:
- Parkinson's disease
- predisposition to gastrointestinal obstruction
- pregnancy
- renal impairment
- severe hepatic impairment.

Breastfeeding is a contraindication.

Quetiapine

❧ Structure
Quetiapine is a dibenzodiazepine derivative. It is available clinically as the quetiapine fumarate salt, with the molecular structure shown in Fig. 3.14.

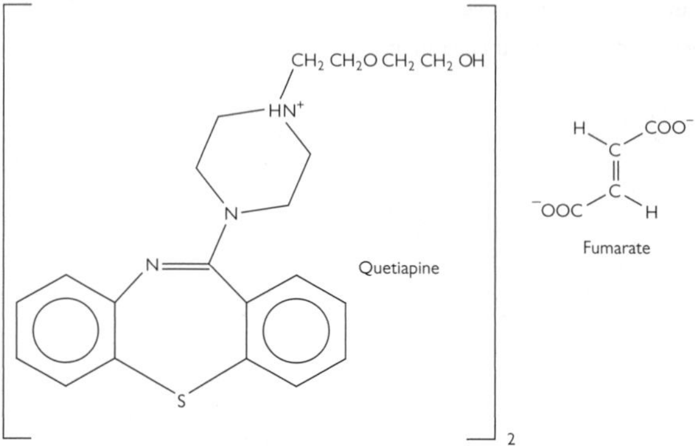

Fig. 3.14 The structure of quetiapine fumarate.

⟳ Receptor binding
Quetiapine has high affinity for:
- histamine H_1 receptors
- α_1-adrenergic receptors
- serotonin 5-HT_2 receptors
- α_2-adrenergic receptors
- dopamine D_2 receptors.

Quetiapine has moderate affinity for:
- serotonin 5-HT_{1A} receptors
- dopamine D_1 receptors.

⚗ Dose
The initiation of quetiapine as an *oral antipsychotic in adults (>18 years) with schizophrenia* should proceed according to the following schedule:
- Day 1: 25mg twice (i.e. 50mg total that day).
- Day 2: 50mg twice (i.e. 100mg total that day).
- Day 3: 100mg twice (i.e. 200mg total that day).
- Day 4: 150mg twice (i.e. 300mg total that day).
- Thereafter: dose adjusted according to clinical response.

The usual maintenance dose of quetiapine is between 300–450mg daily, given as two divided doses (that is, 150 to 225mg twice daily). The maximum total daily dose is 750mg.

In *elderly patients with schizophrenia*, the initiation should proceed as follows:
- Day 1: 25mg once (i.e. 25mg total that day).
- Thereafter: dose increased by 25 to 50mg daily, adjusted according to clinical response, with the total dose being administered in 2 divided doses.

The initiation of quetiapine as an *oral antipsychotic in adults (>18 years) with mania* should proceed according to the following schedule:
- Day 1: 50mg twice (i.e. 100mg total that day).
- Day 2: 100mg twice (i.e. 200mg total that day).
- Day 3: 150mg twice (i.e. 300mg total that day).
- Day 4: 200mg twice (i.e. 400mg total that day).
- Thereafter: dose adjusted according to clinical response in steps of ≤ 200mg daily up to a maximum dose of 800mg daily.

The usual dose range of quetiapine for mania is between 400–800mg daily, given as 2 divided doses (that is, 200–400mg twice daily). The maximum total daily dose is 800mg.

In *elderly patients with mania*, the initiation should proceed as follows:
- Day 1: 25mg once (i.e. 25mg total that day).
- Thereafter: dose increased by 25 to 50mg daily, adjusted according to clinical response, with the total dose being administered in 2 divided doses.

The initiation of quetiapine for the treatment of *depression in adults (>18 years)* should proceed according to the following schedule:
- Day 1: 50mg nocte (i.e. 50mg total that day).
- Day 2: 100mg nocte.
- Day 3: 200mg nocte.
- Day 4: 300mg nocte.
- Thereafter: dose adjusted according to clinical response.

The usual dose range of quetiapine for depression in adults is 300mg nocte. The maximum total daily dose is 600mg.

For maintenance for the prevention of *manic or depressive relapses in bipolar disorder in adults*, the dose of quetiapine is reduced to the lowest effective dose. The range is usually between 300–800mg daily, in 2 divided doses.

A *modified-release form of quetiapine fumarate* is available. The doses differ from those given earlier, as follows.

The initiation of modified-release quetiapine (Seroquel® XL) as an *oral antipsychotic in adults (>18 years) with schizophrenia* should proceed according to the following schedule:
- Day 1: 300mg once.
- Day 2: 600mg once.
- Thereafter: dose adjusted according to clinical response.

The usual maintenance dose of modified-release quetiapine (Seroquel® XL) is 600mg daily, given as one dose. The maximum total daily dose is 800mg, prescribed under specialist supervision.

In *elderly patients with schizophrenia*, the initiation of modified-release quetiapine (Seroquel® XL) should proceed as follows:
- Day 1: 50mg once.
- Thereafter: dose adjusted in steps of 50mg daily, according to clinical response.

The initiation of modified-release quetiapine (Seroquel® XL) as an *oral antipsychotic in adults (>18 years) with mania* should proceed according to the following schedule:
- Day 1: 300mg once.
- Day 2: 600mg once.
- Thereafter: dose adjusted according to clinical response.

The dose range of modified-release quetiapine (Seroquel® XL) for *mania in adults* is between 400–800mg daily, given as one dose daily.

In *elderly patients with mania*, the initiation of modified-release quetiapine (Seroquel® XL) should proceed as follows:
- Day 1: 50mg once.
- Thereafter: dose adjusted in steps of 50mg daily, according to clinical response.

The initiation of modified-release quetiapine (Seroquel® XL) for the treatment of *depression in adults (>18 years)* should proceed according to the following schedule:
- Day 1: 50mg nocte (i.e. 50mg total that day).
- Day 2: 100mg nocte.
- Day 3: 200mg nocte.
- Day 4: 300mg nocte.
- Thereafter: dose adjusted according to clinical response.

The usual dose range of modified-release quetiapine (Seroquel® XL) for *depression in adults* is 300mg nocte. The maximum total daily dose is 600mg.

For maintenance for the prevention of *manic or depressive relapses in bipolar disorder in adults*, the dose of modified-release quetiapine (Seroquel® XL) is reduced to the lowest effective dose. The range is usually between 300–800mg daily, in one daily dose.

The initiation of modified-release quetiapine (Seroquel® XL) for the adjunctive treatment of *depression in adults (>18 years)* should proceed according to the following schedule:
- Day 1: 50mg nocte (i.e. 50mg total that day).
- Day 2: 50mg nocte.
- Day 3: 150mg nocte.
- Day 4: 150mg nocte.
- Thereafter: dose adjusted according to clinical response.

The usual dose range of modified-release quetiapine (Seroquel® XL) for the adjunctive treatment of depression in adults is between 150–300mg daily.

The initiation of modified-release quetiapine (Seroquel® XL) for the adjunctive treatment of *depression in the elderly* should proceed according to the following schedule:
- Day 1: 50mg once daily (e.g. nocte).
- Day 2: 50mg once daily.
- Day 3: 50mg once daily.

- Day 4: if necessary, increase to 100mg once daily.
- Day 5: up to 100mg once daily.
- Day 6: up to 100mg once daily.
- Day 7: up to 100mg once daily.
- Thereafter: dose adjusted according to clinical response in steps of 50mg.

The usual dose range of modified-release quetiapine (Seroquel® XL) for the adjunctive treatment of depression in the elderly is between 50–300mg once daily; a dose of 300mg once daily in the elderly should not be reached before the 22nd day of treatment with this drug.

☺ Side-effects

See the section on side-effects and cautions with antipsychotic drugs, p.71. In addition, the following side-effects may occur:
- asthenia
- blurred vision
- constipation
- drowsiness
- dry mouth
- dysarthria
- dyspepsia
- elevated plasma-cholesterol levels
- elevated plasma-triglyceride levels
- headache
- hyperprolactinaemia
- hypertension
- irritability
- leucopenia
- neutropenia
- peripheral oedema
- rhinitis
- tachycardia.

Less common side-effects include:
- eosinophilia
- restless legs syndrome
- seizures.

Rare side-effects include:
- jaundice
- priapism.

Caution should also be exercised in the following cases:
- cerebrovascular disease
- depressed patients under the age of 25 years (in whom there is an increased risk of suicide)
- hepatic impairment (here the initial adult dose of immediate-release quetiapine should be 25mg daily, increased in daily steps of no higher than 25 to 50mg; for modified-release quetiapine, the initial adult dose should be 50mg daily, increased in steps of no higher than 50mg daily)
- patients at risk of aspiration pneumonia
- pregnancy.
  Breastfeeding is a contraindication.

Risperidone

℘ Structure
Risperidone is a benzisoxazole derivative. Its molecular structure is shown in Fig. 3.15.

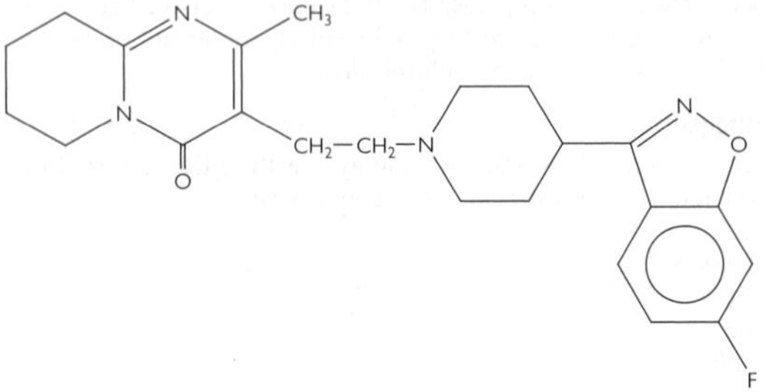

Fig. 3.15 The structure of risperidone.

⟁ Receptor binding
Risperidone has high affinity for:
- dopamine D_2 receptors
- α_1-adrenergic receptors
- α_2-adrenergic receptors
- histamine H_1 receptors.

Risperidone has moderate affinity for:
- serotonin 5-HT_{1C} receptors
- serotonin 5-HT_{1D} receptors
- serotonin 5-HT_{1A} receptors .

Risperidone has low affinity for:
- dopamine D_1 receptors
- haloperidol-sensitive sigma sites.

Risperidone has essentially no affinity for muscarinic or beta-adrenergic receptors.

ⓙ Dose
The initiation of risperidone as an *oral antipsychotic drug in adults (>18 years)* should proceed according to the following schedule:
- Day 1: 2mg in 1–2 divided doses.
- Day 2: 4mg in 1–2 divided doses (but slower titration may be required in some patients).
- Thereafter: 4–6mg daily, with the dose adjusted according to clinical response.

The maximum total daily dose is 16mg, with doses above 10mg daily only to be given if the risk–benefit ratio favours clinical benefit. In elderly patients, and in those with hepatic or renal impairment, the initial dose should be 500 micrograms twice daily (i.e. 1mg total per day). This can be increased by 500 micrograms twice daily (i.e. 1mg total per day) to 1–2mg twice daily (i.e. a total of 2–4mg per day).

The initiation of risperidone as a treatment for *adults (>18 years) with mania* should proceed according to the following schedule:
• Day 1: 2mg in one dose.
• Thereafter: increased if necessary in steps of 1mg daily to a usual dose of 1 to 6mg daily.

In *elderly patients with mania*, the initial dose should be 500 micrograms once daily (i.e. 1mg total per day). This can be increased by 500 micrograms twice daily (i.e. 1mg total per day) to 1–2mg twice daily (i.e. a total of 2 to 4mg per day).

For the treatment of persistent aggression in Alzheimer's disease, the initial dose of risperidone is 250 micrograms twice daily. This can be increased, according to clinical response, in steps of 250 micrograms twice daily on alternate days, up to a usual dose of 500 micrograms twice daily.

In addition to ordinary tablets, oral administration can also be carried out using orodispersible tablets (known as Quicklet®) which dissolve quickly after being placed on the tongue. Their advantages over ordinary tablets are listed in the 'Olanzapine' section, p.81. A liquid preparation is also available for oral administration; it can be diluted in water, black coffee, or orange juice, and should be drunk immediately.

Risperidone is also available in an injectable depot form, which is described in Chapter 4 (p.108).

☺ Side-effects

See the section on side-effects and cautions with antipsychotic drugs, p.71. Relatively common side-effects of risperidone include:
• abdominal pain
• abnormal vision
• agitation
• anxiety
• arthralgia
• asthenia
• constipation
• diarrhoea
• drowsiness
• dry mouth
• dyspepsia
• dyspnoea
• epistaxis
• headache
• myalgia
• nausea
• rash
• sleep disturbance
• tremor
• urinary incontinence
• vomiting.

Less common side-effects include:
- angio-oedema
- anorexia
- blood disorders
- electrocardiographic changes
- hyperprolactinaemia:
  - galactorrhoea
  - gynaecomastia
  - menstrual disturbances
- hypoaesthesia
- impaired concentration
- sexual dysfunction
- tinnitus.

Rare side-effects include:
- abnormal temperature regulation
- hyponatraemia
- intestinal obstruction
- jaundice
- pancreatitis
- seizures.

In addition to those given, caution should also be exercised in the following cases:
- dehydration
- dementia with Lewy bodies
- hepatic impairment (the initial and subsequent oral doses should be halved)
- Parkinson's disease
- pregnancy (risperidone taken during the third trimester is associated with neonatal extrapyramidal effects)
- renal impairment (the initial and subsequent oral doses should be halved).

Contraindications include:
- acute porphyria
- breastfeeding.

Asenapine

This tetracyclic antipsychotic is indicated in the treatment of mania and is therefore considered in Chapter 6 (p.132).

Chapter 4

Antipsychotic depot injections

Administration *96*
Dosage guidelines *99*
Equivalent doses *100*
Choice *101*
Flupentixol decanoate *102*
Fluphenazine decanoate *103*
Haloperidol decanoate *104*
Olanzapine embonate *105*
Paliperidone *106*
Pipotiazine palmitate *107*
Risperidone *108*
Zuclopenthixol decanoate *109*

Administration

Long-acting antipsychotic depot injections may be administered to adults by deep intramuscular injection. They should not be given to children.

Advantages and disadvantages

This form of administration leads to excellent compliance with the medication, as there is slow and sustained absorption of the antipsychotic drug from the depot. Disadvantages of using depot injections include:

- The injections may cause false results from investigations such as the creatine kinase level.
- Extrapyramidal symptoms may occur more often with depot preparations of first-generation antipsychotics than with the corresponding oral preparations. However, depot preparations of second-generation antipsychotics (such as paliperidone and olanzapine embonate), with which such symptoms may be less common, are available.
- They should be used with caution if a patient is taking anticoagulant medication as this may increase the bleeding time.
- General side-effects can include pain, erythema, swelling, nodules, and damage to anatomical structures such as nerves.

Site of injection

The injection of a small volume (maximum 2mL), such as a test dose, using a very small needle can be given into the deltoid muscle in the upper arm. In general, however, with the exception of paliperidone and risperidone (for which the deltoid muscle can be chosen), deep intramuscular injections are given into muscles of the lower limb. There are 2 common choices:

- The buttock. This has the major disadvantage of the possibility of damage to the sciatic nerve. If the buttock is to be used, then ideally the whole buttock should be exposed, the upper and outer quadrant of the buttock thereby identified, and the injection given into this upper outer quadrant (see Fig. 4.1). With a relatively long needle such an injection is more likely to enter the gluteus medius rather than the gluteus maximus. With too short a needle the depot injection is more likely to be deposited in fat rather than muscle. In general, manufacturers of depot antipsychotic medication recommend the gluteal muscles.
- The lateral thigh. The injection is deposited into the vastus lateralis. In general this is safer than trying to inject into the gluteus medius or gluteus maximus. The vastus lateralis is part of the quadriceps femoris; a suitable part of the muscle into which to inject can be found by placing a hand below the greater trochanter of the femur and another hand above the lateral condyle of the femur—the mid-lateral thigh region in between is a suitable area, as shown in Fig. 4.2. (The greater trochanter lies inferior to the middle of the iliac crest, while the lateral femoral condyle is easily felt at the knee, particularly when the knee is flexed.)

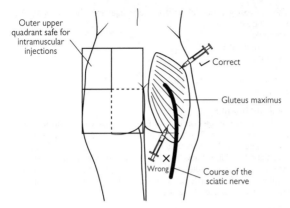

Fig. 4.1 The site of intramuscular injection into the buttock.

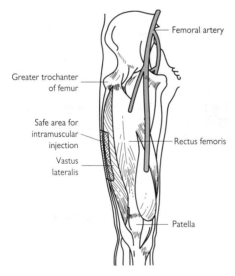

Fig. 4.2 The site of intramuscular injection into the thigh.

When choosing a site for intramuscular injection, the following sites should not be chosen:
- birthmark
- inflammation present
- irritation present
- mole
- oedema present
- scar tissue.

Z-track technique
Normally, the skin in section is as in Fig. 4.3a. The skin is displaced with a finger as in Fig. 4.3b. The needle is then inserted as in Fig. 4.3c, and the depot injected. The needle is then withdrawn. Finally, your finger is removed and the skin returns to its original position as shown in Fig. 4.3d, thereby breaking the needle track and trapping the depot in the muscle without allowing for a ready route of exit of the drug into the subcutaneous tissue or the surface of the skin.

Timing
If the patient has not previously received an injection of the antipsychotic drug, a small test dose should first be given. The frequency of administration of the full depot dose is usually between once per 4 weeks and once per week.

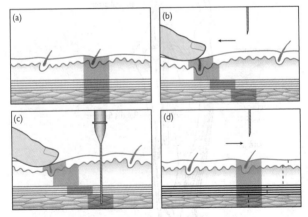

Fig. 4.3 The z-track technique.

Dosage guidelines

The recommendation of the *British National Formulary* is:

'Individual responses to neuroleptic drugs are very variable and to achieve optimum effect, dosage and dosage interval must be titrated according to the patient's response.'

As mentioned in Chapter 3, The Royal College of Psychiatrists have issued the following advice on doses exceeding the *British National Formulary* upper limits (which constitutes unlicensed use).

1. Consider alternative approaches including adjuvant therapy and newer or second-generation antipsychotics such as clozapine.
2. Bear in mind risk factors, including obesity; particular caution is indicated in older patients, especially those over 70.
3. Consider potential for drug interactions.
4. Carry out ECG to exclude untoward abnormalities such as prolonged QT interval; repeat ECG periodically and reduce dose if prolonged QT interval or other adverse abnormality develops.
5. Increase dose slowly and not more often than once weekly.
6. Carry out regular pulse, blood pressure, and temperature checks; ensure that patient maintains adequate fluid intake.
7. Consider high-dose therapy to be for limited period and review regularly; abandon if no improvement after 3 months (return to standard dosage).

In addition, the *British National Formulary* offers the following advice:

'**Important:** When prescribing an antipsychotic for administration on an emergency basis, the intramuscular dose should be **lower** than the corresponding oral dose (owing to absence of first-pass effect), particularly if the patient is very active (increased blood flow to muscle considerably increases the rate of absorption). The prescription should specify the dose for **each route** and should **not** imply that the same dose can be given by mouth or by intramuscular injection. The dose of antipsychotic for emergency use should be reviewed at least **daily**.'

Caution must be exercised in cases of:
• hepatic impairment
• renal impairment.

In such cases, if prescription of an antipsychotic depot is being considered, then reference should be made to the corresponding manufacturer's product literature, and the manufacturer's medical information department may need to be contacted for advice.

In general, these medications are contraindicated in pregnancy.

Equivalent doses

Equivalent doses for a selection of intramuscular depot antipsychotic drugs are given in the *British National Formulary* and reproduced in Table 4.1. Note that these equivalent doses should not be extrapolated beyond the maximum dose for each antipsychotic drug.

Table 4.1 Equivalent doses of depot antipsychotics. Reproduced with kind permission of the Joint Formulary Committee. *British National Formulary*, 51st edn (2006). British Medical Association and Royal Pharmaceutical Society of Great Britain, London.

Antipsychotic	Dose (mg)	Interval
Flupentixol decanoate	40	2 weeks
Fluphenazine decanoate	25	2 weeks
Haloperidol (as decanoate)	100	4 weeks
Pipotiazine palmitate	50	4 weeks
Zuclopenthixol decanoate	200	2 weeks

Choice

As already mentioned, extrapyramidal side-effects are likely to be less common with the use of second-generation antipsychotic preparations than with first-generation depot antipsychotics. For agitation and aggression, zuclopenthixol decanoate may be a particularly good choice.

Flupentixol decanoate

In the UK and USA, flupentixol used to be known as flupenthixol.

⚛ Structure

Flupentixol is a thioxanthene. Its molecular structure is shown in Fig. 3.7 (p.66).

⚗ Dose

The manufacturer recommends deep intramuscular gluteal injection. The adult intramuscular test dose is 20mg. After at least 1 week (7 days), 20–40mg may be given by deep intramuscular injection every 2–4 weeks. The maximum *British National Formulary* dose is 400mg weekly. The doses used in the elderly are initially a quarter to a half of these doses.

Flupentixol decanoate is not recommended for use in children.

☹ Side-effects

As given in Chapter 3 and earlier in this chapter. Flupentixol decanoate may elevate mood.

Fluphenazine decanoate

ࣶ Structure

Fluphenazine is a phenothiazine with a piperazine group attached to the nitrogen-bridge. Its molecular structure is shown in Fig. 4.4.

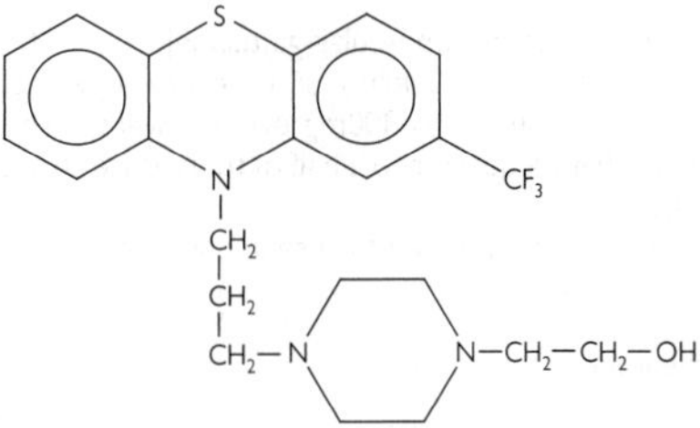

Fig. 4.4 The structure of fluphenazine hydrochloride.

ࣶ Dose

The manufacturer recommends deep intramuscular gluteal injection. The adult intramuscular test dose is 12.5mg, and half of this (6.25mg) in the elderly. After 4–7 days, 12.5–100mg may be given by deep intramuscular injection every 14–35 days.

Fluphenazine decanoate is not recommended for use in children.

☺ Side-effects

As given in Chapter 3 and earlier in this chapter. Although they usually appear within hours, any extrapyramidal side-effects may take longer (days) to manifest. This depot should be avoided in the case of hepatic failure and in the case of renal failure.

Haloperidol decanoate

⚹ Structure

Haloperidol is a butyrophenone. Its molecular structure is shown in Fig. 3.5 (p.63).

⦿ Dose

The manufacturer recommends deep intramuscular gluteal injection. The adult intramuscular antipsychotic dose is initially 50mg every 4 weeks, which may be increased (in 50-mg steps) to 300mg every 4 weeks. The doses used in the elderly are initially a quarter to a half of these doses (that is, 12.5–25mg every 4 weeks).

Haloperidol decanoate is not recommended for use in children.

☺ Side-effects

As given in Chapter 3 and earlier in this chapter.

Olanzapine embonate

⚛ Structure

Olanzapine is a thienobenzodiazepine. Its molecular structure is shown in Fig. 3.13 (p.80).

⚒ Dose

The manufacturer recommends deep intramuscular gluteal injection. It is used for maintenance treatment in adult patients aged between 18–75 years with schizophrenia who tolerate oral olanzapine. The intramuscular depot dosage depends on the oral olanzapine dose that the patient is taking at the time that the depot form is started, as follows:

- If the adult (18–75 years) patient is taking 10mg olanzapine daily, then the initial intramuscular dose of olanzapine embonate is either 210mg every 2 weeks or 405mg every 4 weeks. After 2 months' treatment, the maintenance dose is either 150mg every 2 weeks or 300mg every 4 weeks.
- If the adult (18–75 years) patient is taking 15mg olanzapine daily, then the initial intramuscular dose of olanzapine embonate is 300mg every 2 weeks. After 2 months' treatment, the maintenance dose is either 210mg every 2 weeks or 405mg every 4 weeks.
- If the adult (18–75 years) patient is taking 20mg olanzapine daily, then the initial intramuscular dose of olanzapine embonate is 300mg every 2 weeks. After 2 months' treatment, the maintenance dose is 300mg every 2 weeks.

The manufacturer recommends that the depot dose may be adjusted according to clinical response, up to a maximum of 300mg every 2 weeks. These depot injections are meant to replace the oral olanzapine medication. If patients continue to be prescribed oral olanzapine, then the given doses are too high and the prescribing doctor will need to refer to the manufacturer's product literature.

In the case of either hepatic impairment or renal impairment, smaller doses may be prescribed with caution (initially 150mg every 4 weeks).

☺ Side-effects

As given in Chapter 3 and earlier in this chapter.

Paliperidone

❧ Structure

Paliperidone is 9-hydroxyrisperidone, an active metabolite of risperidone (the molecular structure of which is shown in Fig. 3.15 (p.90).

♪ Dose

The manufacturer recommends deep intramuscular deltoid muscle injection. It is used for maintenance treatment in adult patients with schizophrenia who have previously been responsive to either paliperidone or risperidone. (Such oral antipsychotic medication should be discontinued at the time of initiation of this depot antipsychotic.) The dosing regimen is as follows.

• Day 1: 150mg.
• Day 8 ± 2 (i.e. 1 week later): 100mg.
• Thereafter, a monthly maintenance dose of 75mg (range 50–150mg) into either the deltoid or the gluteal muscle.

The manufacturer recommends that for deltoid administration, a 1½-inch, 22-gauge needle (38.1mm × 0.72mm) be used for patients with a body mass of at least 90kg, while a 1-inch, 23-gauge needle (25.4mm × 0.64mm) should be used for those with a body of less than 90kg. The former size needle should be used for maintenance doses given into the gluteal muscle. The manufacturer also recommends that, to avoid a missed monthly dose, patients may be given the injection up to 7 days before or after the monthly injection due date.

If switching a patient from risperidone depot (Risperdal Consta®) to paliperidone depot (Xeplion®), the latter should be initiated in place of the next scheduled injection of risperidone depot and then continued at monthly intervals.

In the case of mild renal impairment (50mL/min ≤creatinine clearance <80mL/min), the initiation dose of paliperidone depot should be 100mg, followed by a dose of 75mg on day 8; the recommended monthly maintenance dose is 50mg.

This depot is not recommended for use in patients with moderate or severe renal impairment (creatinine clearance <50mL/min). Caution should be exercised in patients suffering from severe hepatic impairment.

☺ Side-effects

As given in Chapter 3 and earlier in this chapter.

Pipotiazine palmitate

Pipotiazine used to be known as pipothiazine.

❧ Structure

Pipotiazine is a phenothiazine with a piperidine ring in the side-chain attached to the nitrogen-bridge. Its molecular structure is shown in Fig. 4.5.

♪ Dose

The manufacture recommends deep intramuscular gluteal injection. The adult intramuscular test dose is 25mg. After 4–7 days, 25–50mg may be given. The maintenance dose usually falls between 50–100mg every 4 weeks. The maximum *British National Formulary* dose is 200mg every 4 weeks. The doses used in the elderly are initially 5–10mg.

Pipotiazine palmitate is not recommended for use in children.

As mentioned in Chapter 3 and earlier in this chapter, caution must be exercised in hepatic impairment and renal impairment, and also, in the case of this depot, in patients suffering from thyrotoxicosis or hypothyroidism. It should preferably be avoided in pregnancy and during breast-feeding.

☺ Side-effects

See the details given earlier in this chapter and in Chapter 3.

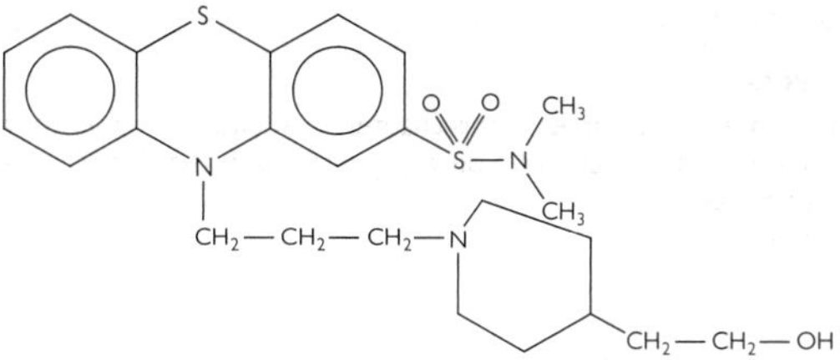

Fig. 4.5 The structure of pipotiazine.

Risperidone

⚘ Structure

Risperidone is a benzisoxazole derivative. Its molecular structure is shown in Fig. 3.15 (p.90).

⚗ Dose

The manufacture recommends deep intramuscular deltoid or gluteal injection. The depot is indicated in adult patients (>18 years) with schizophrenia or other psychoses who are tolerant to oral risperidone. The initial adult intramuscular dose varies depending on the dose of oral risperidone being taken at the time:

- Oral risperidone dose ≤4mg per day: start on 25mg intramuscular risperidone every 2 weeks; oral risperidone may be continued for 4–6 weeks
- Oral risperidone dose >4mg per day: start on 37.5mg intramuscular risperidone every 2 weeks; oral risperidone may be continued for 4–6 weeks.

The dose may be increased by 12.5mg every 4 weeks up to a maximum of 50mg every 2 weeks. Oral risperidone may be required during adjustment of the risperidone depot dose.

Depot injections of risperidone are not recommended for use in those under the age of 18 years.

☺ Side-effects

As given in Chapter 3 and earlier in this chapter. In addition, the following relatively common side-effects have been reported with the depot long-acting form of risperidone:

- hypertension
- depression
- paraesthesia.

Less common side-effects of depot risperidone, additional to those already mentioned in Chapter 3 and earlier in this chapter, include:

- apathy
- injection-site reactions
- pruritus
- weight decrease.

Zuclopenthixol decanoate

℞ Structure
Zuclopenthixol is a thioxanthene. Its molecular structure, shown in Fig. 3.8 (p.68), is similar to that of flupentixol (see Fig. 3.7, p.66), which is also a thioxanthene.

💉 Dose
The manufacturer recommends deep intramuscular injection into the upper outer buttock or the lateral thigh. The adult intramuscular test dose is 100mg. After at least 1 week (7 days), 200–500mg may be given by deep intramuscular injection every 1–4 weeks. The maximum *British National Formulary* dose is 600mg weekly. The doses used in the elderly are initially a quarter to a half of the usual adult starting dose.

Zuclopenthixol decanoate is not recommended for use in children.

☺ Side-effects
As given in Chapter 3 and earlier in this chapter.

It should be avoided in patients with acute porphyria and it should not be used at the same time as drugs that prolong the QT interval; zuclopenthixol decanoate should be used with caution in patients who have prolonged QT intervals.

Zuclopenthixol decanoate

Structure

Dose

Side-effects

Treatment-resistant schizophrenia

Treatment-resistant schizophrenia *112*

Treatment-resistant schizophrenia

In 2009, NICE published the following guidance for the treatment of patients suffering from schizophrenia who have not responded adequately to treatment.

- 'For people with schizophrenia whose illness has not responded adequately to pharmacological or psychological treatment:
  - review the diagnosis
  - establish that there has been adherence to antipsychotic medication, prescribed at an adequate dose and for the correct duration
  - review engagement with and use of psychological treatments and ensure that these have been offered according to this guideline. If family intervention has been undertaken suggest CBT [cognitive behavioural therapy]; if CBT has been undertaken suggest family intervention for people in close contact with their families
  - consider other causes of non-response, such as comorbid substance misuse (including alcohol), the concurrent use of other prescribed medication or physical illness.
- Offer clozapine to people with schizophrenia whose illness has not responded adequately to treatment despite the sequential use of adequate doses of at least two different antipsychotic drugs. At least one of the drugs should be a non-clozapine second-generation antipsychotic.'

Antimanic drugs

The use of antimanic drugs *114*
Treatment strategies for bipolar I disorder *115*
Lithium salts *116*
Carbamazepine *122*
Valproic acid *128*
Second-generation antipsychotics *130*
Asenapine *132*

The use of antimanic drugs

The antimanic drugs considered in this chapter are lithium salts, carba-mazepine, and semisodium valproate (containing valproic acid). Lithium carbonate and lithium citrate are particularly useful in the prophylaxis of bipolar mood disorder, as well as having a role in the treatment of mania itself. The antiepileptic drug carbamazepine may be used as an alternative to lithium salts in the prophylaxis of bipolar mood disorder in patients who do not respond to lithium salts, particularly in those who are rapid cyclers suffering at least 4 relapses (mania or depression) per year. Valproic acid (semisodium valproate) is an effective treatment for mania in many cases of bipolar disorder.

Two other groups of drugs may also be used in the treatment of mania, namely benzodiazepines and antipsychotic drugs.

Benzodiazepines, which are briefly discussed in Chapter 12, can be used in the short-term treatment of the initial symptoms of mania, but should not be used long-term as they are associated with a risk of dependency.

In general, antipsychotic drugs act more rapidly than lithium salts in the treatment of mania or hypomania. (One patient is reported to have drawn the analogy that acute mania was like being in an-out-of-control car, with antipsychotic drugs acting as if pressure were being applied to the brake pedal, whereas lithium therapy felt more like the effect of adjusting the accelerator pedal.) In mild to moderate mania it may be better to treat with lithium or another mood stabilizer (such as valproic acid) alone, owing to their specific antimanic action and also in order to reduce the level of side-effects.

The novel antipsychotic asenapine has recently become available for bipolar I disorder.

Treatment strategies for bipolar I disorder

Maron and Young (2011) have suggested the treatment strategies for bipolar I disorder shown in Table 6.1.

Table 6.1 Treatment strategies for bipolar I disorder. Reproduced from Maron and Young (2011).

Acute mania
- Stop antidepressant treatment
- Consider antipsychotics or mood stabilizers
- Combine antipsychotic and valproate or lithium if response is inadequate
- Monitor compliance, dose, and plasma level (lithium, valproate)
- Consider adding short-term benzodiazepine
- Consider electroconvulsive therapy if refractory state

Depressive episode
- Consider quetiapine monotherapy
- Consider lithium and lamotrigine combination
- Consider olanzapine and fluoxetine combination
- Consider adding antidepressants
- Consider electroconvulsive therapy if refractory state

Prophylaxis
- Consider lithium, valproate, quetiapine, or olanzapine as first-line prophylactic agents
- Continue treatment for at least 2 years
- Consider SSRI or cognitive behavioural therapy with a mood stabilizer or quetiapine for chronic recurrent depression
- Combine lithium and valproate for the prophylaxis of rapid cycling illness

Lithium salts

The lithium salts most commonly used in clinical psychiatric practice are:
- Lithium carbonate (e.g. Camcolit®, Liskonum®, and Priadel®)
- Lithium citrate (e.g. Li-Liquid® and Priadel® liquid).

℘ Structure

The active ingredient of lithium salts is the lithium ion, Li⁺. Lithium is an element, in the same group in the periodic table as the metals sodium, potassium, and rubidium. It has the atomic number 3 and an atomic mass of 6.941.

Indications

Circumstances in which lithium salts are used include the:
- prophylaxis of bipolar mood disorder
- treatment of mania or hypomania
- treatment of resistant depression
- prophylaxis of recurrent depression
- treatment of aggression
- treatment of self-mutilation.

Contraindications and cautions

Lithium therapy should not be used in the following conditions:
- Cardiac failure.
- Renal impairment.
- Other conditions associated with sodium ion imbalance, such as
  - primary hypoadrenalism (Addison's disease)
  - congenital adrenal hyperplasia
  - corticosterone methyl oxidase deficiency types I and II
  - hyporeninaemic hypoaldosteronism
  - pseudohypoaldosteronism type I
  - Barrter's syndrome
  - following renal transplantation
  - following relief of urinary tract obstruction
  - acute interstitial nephritis.
- Pregnancy—if at all possible, lithium therapy should be avoided in pregnancy, as lithium is associated with a risk of teratogenicity.

Lithium should be stopped or the dose reduced (with careful monitoring of fluid balance and electrolytes) in the following conditions:
- diarrhoea
- vomiting
- intercurrent infection—particularly if profuse sweating occurs.

Lithium should be used with caution in the following conditions:
- lactation
- myasthenia gravis.

It is not recommended that lithium be used in childhood, while a reduced dose should be used in the elderly. While lithium therapy may be continued during minor surgery, so long as fluid balance and electrolytes are monitored carefully, in general lithium should be stopped 24 hours before major surgery.

How to use lithium salts

Being an element, lithium (actually, Li^+ cations) are not metabolized but are excreted mainly by the kidneys. Given that lithium has a narrow therapeutic index (see 'Monitoring', p.119), it is necessary to carry out tests of renal function before initiating treatment with lithium. In most patients this involves checking the plasma urea, electrolytes, and creatinine levels. If, however, there is an indication of poor renal function, then full renal function studies need to be carried out before starting lithium treatment.

Lithium salts are administered orally at a dose that leads to a serum lithium ion concentration of between 0.4–1mmol/L 12 hours after the last dose, 4–7 days after the initiation of treatment.

Different lithium preparations vary in the bioavailability, and therefore it is recommended that if the preparation is to be changed, then the serum lithium ion concentration precautions should be taken again.

After dosage stabilization, the lithium salt may be given once daily rather than in divided doses, although there are no hard and fast rules. Those who administer it once daily often prefer to give the daily dose at night, in order to reduce the impact of side-effects.

For patients in whom compliance is problematic, and for those suffering from dysphagia, an oral solution and a liquid preparation of lithium citrate are available as alternatives to tablets of lithium carbonate or lithium citrate. Note that 200mg lithium carbonate is the bioequivalent of 509mg lithium citrate, in respect of lithium.

The manufacturers' dosage recommendations are as follows.

Camcolit®

- Serum monitoring should be carried out (see 'Monitoring', p.119).
- For treatment, initially start with 1–1.5g daily.
- For prophylaxis, initially start with 300–400mg daily.
- It is not recommended for use in children.

Liskonum®

- Serum monitoring should be carried out (see 'Monitoring', p.119).
- For treatment, initially start with 450–675mg twice daily; 225mg twice daily in the elderly.
- For prophylaxis, initially start with 450mg twice daily; 225mg twice daily in the elderly.
- It is not recommended for use in children.

Priadel® tablets

- Serum monitoring should be carried out (see 'Monitoring', p.119).
- For treatment, initially start with 0.4–1.2g daily as a single dose or in 2 divided doses; 400mg daily in the elderly and in patients weighing less than 50kg.
- For prophylaxis, initially start with 0.4–1.2g daily as a single dose or in 2 divided doses; 400mg daily in the elderly and in patients weighing less than 50kg.
- It is not recommended for use in children.

Priadel® liquid

- Plasma monitoring should be carried out (see 'Monitoring', p.119).
- For treatment, initially start with 1.04–3.12g daily in 2 divided doses; 520mg twice daily in the elderly and in patients weighing less than 50kg.
- For prophylaxis, initially start with 1.04–3.12g daily in 2 divided doses; 520mg twice daily in the elderly and in patients weighing less than 50kg.
- It is not recommended for use in children.

Li-Liquid® (oral solution)

- Plasma monitoring should be carried out (see 'Monitoring', p.119).
- For treatment, initially start with 1.018–3.054 g daily in 2 divided doses; 509mg twice daily in the elderly and in patients weighing less than 50kg.
- For prophylaxis, initially start with 1.018–3.054 g daily in 2 divided doses; 509mg twice daily in the elderly and in patients weighing less than 50kg.
- It is not recommended for use in children.

☺ Side-effects

The side-effects of lithium include:
- gastrointestinal disturbances
- renal impairment:
  - polyuria
  - impaired urinary concentration
- polydipsia
- dry mouth
- metallic taste
- weight gain
- oedema
- fatigue
- fine tremor.

Note that oedema should *not* be treated with diuretics, since thiazide and loop diuretics reduce lithium excretion and so may cause lithium intoxication; oedema may respond to a reduction in the daily lithium dose.

Lithium intoxication

Signs of lithium intoxication are:
- blurred vision
- increasing gastrointestinal disturbances:
  - anorexia
  - vomiting
  - diarrhoea
- muscle weakness
- mild drowsiness and sluggishness progressing to giddiness with ataxia
- lack of coordination
- tinnitus
- dysarthria
- nystagmus
- renal impairment
- coarse tremor.

Lithium treatment should be stopped immediately under these circumstances. The serum lithium ion concentration should be re-checked and appropriate steps taken to reverse the toxicity.

Severe overdosage

At serum lithium ion concentrations of greater than 2mmol/L, the following effects occur:
- hyperreflexia and hyperextension of the limbs
- toxic psychoses
- convulsions
- syncope
- electrolyte imbalance
- dehydration
- hypotension
- oliguria
- circulatory failure
- renal failure
- coma
- death.

This is a medical emergency requiring urgent inpatient admission and treatment. The treatment is supportive, with attention to electrolyte balance and renal function. Convulsions should be controlled. If there is renal failure, haemodialysis may be required. If the severe overdosage has resulted from the ingestion of large amounts of lithium salts, then bowel irrigation should be considered; in any event, the advice of a poisons information centre should be sought.

Long-term treatment

Side-effects following long-term treatment with lithium include:
- thyroid function disturbances:
  - goitre
  - hypothyroidism
- memory impairment
- nephrotoxicity
- cardiovascular changes:
  - T-wave flattening on the ECG
  - arrhythmias.

Monitoring

The therapeutic index of lithium is low. (This is the ratio of the toxic dose to the therapeutic dose.) Hence, regular monitoring needs to take place of serum lithium ion concentrations. Indeed, lithium should not be prescribed if such monitoring facilities are not available. Serum levels are determined 12 hours after an oral dose, and the dose is adjusted to achieve a serum lithium ion concentration of 0.4–1.0mmol/L. The lower levels of this range are required for maintenance therapy and for the elderly.

After the serum level determination(s) at the time of lithium initiation described here (to achieve a serum lithium ion concentration of between 0.4–1mmol/L 12 hours after the last dose, 4–7 days after the initiation of treatment), serum lithium ion concentrations should be determined every week until the lithium dose has remained constant for 4 consecutive weeks. After that, it should be monitored every 3 months.

It is good practice to check the plasma urea, electrolytes, and creatinine levels at the same time as the lithium levels, in order to monitor renal function.

As thyroid function disturbances are a recognized long-term side-effect of lithium therapy, it is also good clinical practice to carry out thyroid function tests every 6 months, beginning with a baseline test at the time of initiation of lithium therapy.

What to tell the patient

In view of the side-effects of lithium, and its narrow therapeutic to toxic ratio (low therapeutic index), patients should be given a lithium card. The lithium card:

• Describes the side-effects of lithium therapy.
• Explains to the patient how they should take their lithium treatment.
• Emphasizes the need for regular blood checks.

It is important to explain to the patient that he/she should maintain an adequate fluid intake; this is particularly important in hot weather or during bouts of prolonged physical exertion. The patient should also be asked to avoid dietary changes that might significantly alter their intake of sodium (e.g. from common salt, as in salty foods, or from monosodium glutamate, as in Chinese take-away meals).

Carbamazepine

Carbamazepine was first introduced clinically (in the 1960s) as a treatment for epilepsy.

♽ Structure

Carbamazepine is an iminostilbene derivative which is related in structure to that of tricyclic antidepressants, as shown in Fig. 6.1.

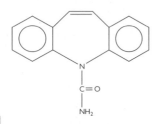

Fig. 6.1 The structure of carbamazepine.

♪ Dose

The initial dose of carbamazepine as an oral drug used in the prophylaxis of bipolar mood disorder in adults is 400mg daily, administered in divided doses. This can be increased, according to clinical response, up to a usual range of between 400–600mg daily. The *British National Formulary* maximum total daily dose is 1600mg (1.6g). In the elderly, the initial dose should be reduced.

Carbamazepine levels in the plasma can be measured by most hospital laboratories in the UK. While a plasma concentration of between 4–12mg/L is considered to be optimum for its antiepileptic action, plasma concentrations are probably not particularly helpful when using carbamazepine in the prophylaxis of bipolar mood disorder, except that central nervous system side-effects are more likely once the plasma concentration exceeds 9mg/L.

Owing to the potential adverse actions of carbamazepine on the blood (see 'Side-effects', p.123), it is prudent to measure the full blood count before initiating treatment with this drug and also to monitor the full blood count regularly during treatment with it.

Baseline and regular monitoring of liver function tests should also be carried out, owing to the potential for carbamazepine to cause hepatic damage (see 'Side-effects', p.123). This is particularly important in the case of patients who have a history of liver disease.

Ideally, baseline and regular ocular examinations should also be carried out, in view of the possibility of ocular changes following treatment with carbamazepine (see 'Side-effects', p.123). These examinations should ideally include slit-lamp investigations, fundoscopy, and tonometry.

Baseline and regular monitoring of renal function, including full urinalysis, should be carried out, since carbamazepine treatment is associated with renal dysfunction.

Note that pharmacotherapy with carbamazepine may be associated with:
• hyponatraemia (which can lead to water intoxication)
• changes in thyroid function tests
• interference with some pregnancy tests.

☻ Side-effects

Pharmacotherapy with carbamazepine is associated with a 5–8-fold increase in the risk of developing aplastic anaemia and agranulocytosis. Transient or persistent decreased platelet counts and/or white blood cell counts may occur, although it is not known what the risk is of these progressing to aplastic anaemia or agranulocytosis. Serious consideration should be given to stopping treatment with carbamazepine if the patient develops leucopenia, thrombocytopenia, agranulocytosis, aplastic anaemia, or another blood disorder. (As mentioned earlier, the full blood count should ideally be monitored regularly while being treated with carbamazepine.)

Relatively common side-effects of carbamazepine, particularly in the initial treatment phase, include:
• blood disorder:
  • eosinophilia
  • leucopenia
  • thrombocytopenia
  • haemolytic anaemia
  • aplastic anaemia
• dizziness
• dermatitis
• urticaria
• drowsiness
• dry mouth
• oedema
• ataxia
• fatigue
• headache
• unsteadiness
• nausea
• vomiting.

Starting carbamazepine treatment at low dosages (see p.122) may reduce the chances of these initial side-effects occurring.

Carbamazepine may affect the following systems:
• haemopoietic—see earlier in section
• skin:
  • pruritic and erythematous rashes (carbamazepine should be withdrawn if the erythematous rashes worsen or are accompanied by other symptoms or signs)
  • urticaria
  • toxic epidermal necrolysis (Lyell's syndrome)
  • Stevens–Johnson syndrome
  • photosensitivity reactions
  • pigmentation changes

- exfoliative dermatitis
- erythema multiforme
- erythema nodosum
- purpura
- aggravation of systemic lupus erythematosus
- alopecia
- diaphoresis
- possibly hirsutism
- cardiovascular:
  - congestive cardiac failure
  - oedema
  - aggravation of hypertension
  - hypotension
  - syncope and collapse
  - aggravation of coronary artery disease
  - arrhythmias
  - atrioventricular (AV) block
  - thrombophlebitis
  - thromboembolism
- immune:
  - lymphadenopathy
- hepatic:
  - abnormal liver function tests
  - cholestatic jaundice
  - hepatocellular jaundice
  - hepatitis
  - hepatic failure (very rare)
- pancreas:
  - pancreatitis
- respiratory:
  - pulmonary hypersensitivity (with pyrexia, dyspnoea, pneumonitis or pneumonia)
- genitourinary:
  - urinary frequency
  - proteinuria
  - acute urinary retention
  - oliguria with raised blood pressure
  - azotaemia
  - renal failure
  - impotence
  - impaired fertility
  - albuminuria
  - glycosuria
  - microscopic deposits in the urine
- digestive:
  - nausea
  - vomiting
  - gastric distress and abdominal pain
  - diarrhoea
  - constipation

- anorexia
- dry mouth
- dry pharynx
- glossitis
- stomatitis
- breasts:
  - galactorrhoea
  - gynaecomastia
- nervous:
  - dizziness
  - drowsiness
  - disturbances of coordination
  - headache
  - fatigue
  - blurred vision
  - visual hallucinations
  - transient diplopia (often associated with peak plasma concentrations)
  - oculomotor disturbances
  - nystagmus
  - speech disturbances
  - dyskinesias
  - peripheral neuritis
  - paraesthesia
  - depression (with agitation)
  - aggression
  - activation of psychosis
  - tinnitus
  - hyperacusis
  - neuroleptic malignant syndrome (rare)
- ocular:
  - punctuate cortical lens opacities
  - conjunctivitis
- musculoskeletal:
  - arthralgia
  - muscle aches
  - leg cramps
  - bone metabolism disturbances (with osteomalacia)
- metabolism:
  - pyrexia and chills
  - syndrome of inappropriate antidiuretic hormone (ADH) secretion
  - frank water intoxication (with hyponatraemia)
  - hypocalcaemia
- others:
  - multiorgan hypersensitivity reactions (days to months after commencing carbamazepine treatment)—symptoms and signs may include pyrexia, skin rashes, vasculitis, lymphadenopathy, disorders that mimic lymphoma, arthralgia, leucopenia, eosinophilia, hepatosplenomegaly, abnormal liver function tests; affected organs

- may include the liver, skin, immune system, lungs, kidneys, pancreas, myocardium and colon
- a systemic lupus erythematosus (SLE)-type syndrome
- raised levels of cholesterol, high-density lipoprotein cholesterol and triglycerides
- suppository-related rectal irritation
- asceptic meningitis (very rare).

Caution should also be exercised in the following cases:
- hepatic impairment
- renal impairment
- cardiac disease
- skin reactions
- history of haematological reactions to other drugs
- glaucoma
- pregnancy
- breastfeeding.

Contraindications are:
- AV conduction abnormalities (unless the patient is artificially paced)
- history of bone marrow depression
- acute porphyria.

Valproic acid

Valproic acid (as semisodium valproate) is licensed in the UK for treating manic episodes associated with bipolar disorder, and it may also be useful in lithium-resistant bipolar patients. It should not be confused with the related antiepileptic and antimigraine drug sodium valproate. In some countries, semisodium valproate is also known as divalproex sodium.

Structure

Semisodium valproate is sodium hydrogen bis(2-propylpentanoate). It consists of a stable coordination compound of sodium valproate and valproic acid in a one-to-one molar ratio, as shown in Fig. 6.2.

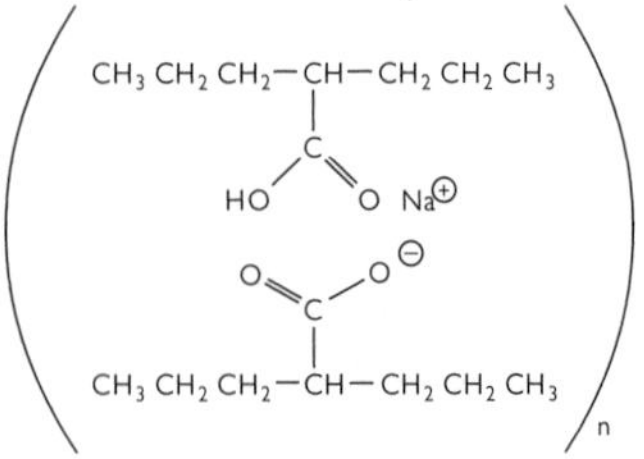

Fig. 6.2 The structure of semisodium valproate.

Dose

The initial adult dose of valproic acid (semisodium valproate) as an oral drug for the treatment of manic episodes associated with bipolar disorder is 750mg daily in 2–3 divided doses. This can be increased, according to clinical response, to between 1–2g (1000–2000mg) daily.

A reduced starting dose of no more than 250mg daily should be used in the elderly as there is a reduction in unbound clearance of valproic acid and a possibility of greater sensitivity to somnolence in this age group. Dosage increases should be only very gradual in this age group, with regular monitoring of fluid intake, nutritional intake, dehydration, somnolence, and other side-effects.

Valproic acid is not recommended for use in those under the age of 18 years.

Side-effects

Relatively common side-effects include:
- gastrointestinal system:
  - nausea
  - gastric irritation
  - diarrhoea
- hyperammonaemia
- thrombocytopenia
- transient hair loss.

Less common (but not rare) side-effects include:

- increased alertness
- aggression
- hyperactivity
- other behavioural disturbances
- ataxia
- tremor
- vasculitis.

Incidents of fatal hepatic failure in patients treated with this drug have occurred; the first 6 months of treatment appear to be the time of particular risk. Therefore, liver function and symptoms and signs of liver failure should be monitored before starting pharmacotherapy with semisodium valproate and during the first 6 months of treatment. Note that hyperammonaemia may occur in spite of normal liver function test results. Hyperammonaemic encephalopathy should be considered in patients who develop unexplained lethargy and vomiting or unexplained adverse changes in mental state. Cases of fatal hyperammonaemic encephalopathy have occurred in patients with urea cycle disorders (particularly ornithine transcarbamylase deficiency) following initiation of treatment with this drug.

Platelet counts and coagulation tests should be carried out at before starting treatment and at regular intervals. Semisodium valproate has been associated with thrombocytopenia, inhibition of the secondary phase of platelet aggregation, low fibrinogen, etc.

Semisodium valproate treatment may be associated with alterations in thyroid function tests. It may also be associated with false-positive urinary ketone testing (valproic acid is partially eliminated as a keto-metabolite in the urine).

The drug treatment should be withdrawn only gradually.

Caution should be exercised in the following cases:

- patients undergoing surgery—ensure that their bleeding time is not unduly impaired beforehand
- renal impairment
- pregnancy
- breastfeeding
- SLE.

Contraindications include:

- active liver disease
- family history of severe hepatic dysfunction
- acute porphyria
- urea cycle disorders.

For patients who have little exposure of their skin to sunlight or poor dietary calcium intake, or who are chronically immobilized, nutritional supplementation vitamin D should be considered.

Patients and their relatives and carers should be given advice on how to recognize symptoms and signs of liver failure, hyperammonaemia, pancreatitis and blood disorders. They should be told to seek urgent medical advice if the patient appears to be developing any of these potentially fatal disorders.

Second-generation antipsychotics

These are considered in Chapters 3 and 4. There is particularly good evidence in favour of the use of quetiapine in bipolar I disorder (see Table 6.1, p.115); this can be a lower dose than that used in the pharmacotherapy of schizophrenia.

Asenapine

This new sublingually administered antipsychotic drug has been introduced (in 2012 in the UK) for the treatment of moderate to severe manic episodes in bipolar I disorder in adults.

⅋ Structure

Asenapine has a novel molecular structure that is not related to that of any existing second-generation antipsychotic drug. Its tetracyclic structure is shown in Fig. 6.3.

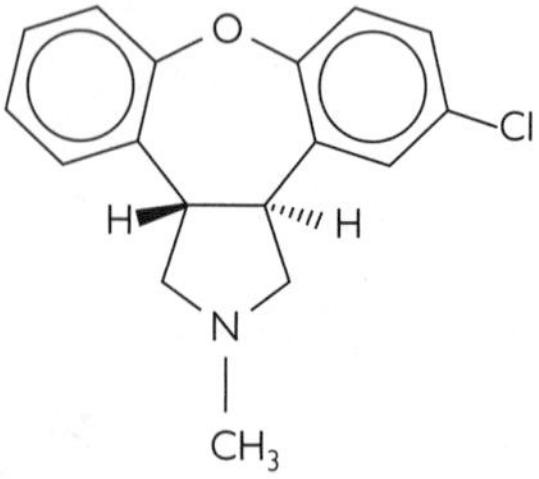

Fig. 6.3 The structure of asenapine.

⊕ Receptor binding

Asenapine has high affinity for:

- α_{2B}-adrenergic receptors
- serotonin 5-HT$_{2A}$ receptors
- serotonin 5-HT$_{2B}$ receptors
- serotonin 5-HT$_{2C}$ receptors
- serotonin 5-HT$_6$ receptors
- serotonin 5-HT$_7$ receptors
- dopamine D$_3$ receptors.

There is little binding to muscarinic receptors. The strong antagonism to 5-HT$_6$ and 5-HT$_7$ receptors may lead to cognitive, antianxiety, and mood stabilization beneficial actions, while the poor binding to muscarinic receptors means that antimuscarinic side-effects are likely to be low. The receptor binding characteristics are also likely to translate into a low level of adverse movement side-effects.

♪ Dose

For adults (aged between 18–65 years) suffering from a manic episode, the starting dose as monotherapy is 10mg twice daily, taken as one dose in the morning and one in the evening. This can be adjusted downwards to 5mg twice daily, according to clinical response. For combination therapy, the recommended starting dose is 5mg twice daily, and according to clinical response this may be increased to 10mg twice daily.

The formulation of asenapine maleate is as sublingual tablets. A tablet is placed under the tongue, where it dissolves. A tablet should neither be chewed nor swallowed. If being taken with other medication, then the asenapine sublingual tablet should be taken last. The patient should also avoid eating or drinking for at least 10 minutes after taking asenapine sublingually.

☹ Side-effects

Relatively common side-effects include:

- somnolence
- anxiety
- weight gain
- increased appetite
- dystonia
- akathisia
- dyskinesia
- parkinsonism
- sedation
- dizziness
- dysgeusia
- oral hypoaesthesia
- increased alanine aminotransferase
- muscle rigidity
- fatigue.

It is probably safest if, in general, patients are advised not to drive a car or operate machinery. Asenapine is not recommended for the treatment of patients with dementia-related psychosis. It should be used with caution in moderate hepatic impairment. It should be discontinued if symptomatology indicative of neuroleptic malignant syndrome appear, and it should probably be discontinued if tardive dyskinesia appears to be developing.

Contraindications include:

- severely impaired hepatic function
- hypersensitivity to the active substance or to excipients
- pregnancy
- breastfeeding.

Tricyclic and related antidepressant drugs

The use of tricyclic antidepressants *136*
Dosage *137*
Choice *138*
Withdrawal *140*
Driving and the use of machinery *141*
Amitriptyline *142*
Imipramine *145*
Trimipramine *146*
Dosulepin *147*
Clomipramine *148*
Lofepramine *149*
Nortriptyline *150*
Doxepin *151*
Trazodone *152*
Mianserin *153*

The use of tricyclic antidepressants

Ever since Kuhn (1958) discovered the antidepressive actions of the archetypal tricyclic antidepressant imipramine, tricyclic antidepressants and related drugs have played an important part in the pharmacotherapy of depression. It was not until the 1980s, with the advent of SSRIs (see Chapter 9) that tricyclic antidepressants and related drugs began to be displaced from their position as the first-line pharmacological treatment for depression. In addition to their use in the treatment of depression, various tricyclic antidepressants are also used in the pharmacotherapy of dysthymia, panic disorder, phobic and obsessional states, childhood nocturnal enuresis, neuralgia, pruritus in eczema, and as an adjunctive treatment of cataplexy associated with narcolepsy.

Dosage

In general, tricyclic antidepressants have long half-lives. This allows for clinically effective once-daily dosing. It may be best to give more sedating antidepressants, such as amitriptyline, as a once-daily bedtime dose, to aid sleep, and to give less sedating ones, such as imipramine, earlier in the day, perhaps even first thing in the morning.

The elderly are particularly vulnerable to the hypotensive and hyponatraemic actions of tricyclic antidepressants. For these reasons, the initial dosage used in elderly patients should be kept low.

Choice

The tricyclic antidepressants include:
- dibenzocycloheptanes:
  - amitriptyline
  - nortriptyline
- iminodibenzyls:
  - clomipramine
  - imipramine
  - trimipramine
- others:
  - dosulepin (dothiepin)
  - doxepin
  - lofepramine.

Tricyclic antidepressant-related antidepressants include:
- trazodone.

Tetracyclic antidepressants include:
- mianserin.

The more sedative tricyclic and related antidepressants include:
- amitriptyline
- clomipramine
- dosulepin
- doxepin
- mianserin
- trazodone
- trimipramine.

These are more appropriate for patients suffering from agitation, anxiety, and, if given at bedtime, insomnia.
    The less sedative tricyclic and related antidepressants include:
- imipramine
- lofepramine
- nortriptyline.

These are more appropriate for patients suffering from withdrawal or apathy.
    The *British National Formulary* (62nd edition) makes the following important comments on these different antidepressants:

Overdosage Limited quantities of tricyclic antidepressants should be prescribed at any one time because their cardiovascular and epileptogenic effects are dangerous in overdosage. In particular, overdosage with dosulepin and amitriptyline is associated with a relatively high rate of fatality. Lofepramine is associated with the lowest risk of fatality in overdosage, in comparison with other tricyclic antidepressant drugs....

Tricyclic and related antidepressants...have varying degrees of antimuscarinic side-effects and cardiotoxicity in overdosage, which may be important in individual patients. **Lofepramine** has a lower incidence of side-effects and is less dangerous in overdosage but is infrequently associated with hepatic toxicity. **Imipramine** is also well established, but has more marked antimuscarinic side-effects than other tricyclic and related antidepressants. **Amitriptyline** and **dosulepin** are effective but they are particularly dangerous in overdosage (see 'Overdosage', p.138) and are not recommended for the treatment of depression; dosulepin should only be prescribed by specialists.'

Withdrawal

Withdrawal of pharmacotherapy of drugs in this group should, as far as is possible, take place gradually.

Driving and the use of machinery

Most tricyclic antidepressants seriously impair driving performance, even more so than alcohol or benzodiazepines; in contrast SSRIs do not do so (Hale, 1994). Ramaekers (2003) reviewed the major results from studies published between 1983 and 2000 that examined the effects of antidepressants on actual driving performance using a standard test. Adverse changes on that test after acute doses of amitriptyline, imipramine, doxepin, and mianserin were comparable to those seen in drivers conducting this test with a blood alcohol level of at least 0.8mg/mL. Given the potential hazard of these drugs for driving, patients should not drive while taking them. They should also be strongly advised not to operate dangerous machinery.

Amitriptyline

As mentioned earlier, amitriptyline is particularly dangerous in overdosage and is not recommended for the treatment of depression. Details of its structure and side-effects are given here for comparison with other tricyclic and related antidepressants.

⅋ Structure
The tricyclic structure of amitriptyline is shown in Fig. 7.1.

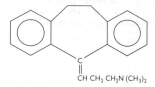

Fig. 7.1 The structure of amitriptyline.

☹ Side-effects
Tricyclic antidepressants are believed to achieve their antidepressant activity through the following postulated actions:
• inhibition of re-uptake of noradrenaline
• inhibition of re-uptake of serotonin (5-HT).

This is the reason that tricyclic antidepressants are known as monoamine re-uptake inhibitors (or MARIs for short). The antiadrenergic action gives rise to the side-effect of postural hypotension, to which, as mentioned here, elderly patients are particularly susceptible. The action on serotonin re-uptake gives rise to gastrointestinal side-effects such as nausea and vomiting.

Tricyclic antidepressants also have antimuscarinic (anticholinergic) actions. These cause antimuscarinic side-effects, including:
• dry mouth
• blurred vision
• mydriasis
• drowsiness
• disturbance of accommodation
• increased intraocular pressure
• urinary retention
• dilatation of the urinary tract
• constipation
• paralytic ileus
• hyperpyrexia.

Other side-effects, given by body systems, include:
• cardiovascular:
  • ECG changes
  • AV conduction changes

- arrhythmias
- postural hypotension
- tachycardia
- palpitations
- syncope
- heart block
- myocardial infarction and stroke have been reported with tricyclic antidepressants
- nervous and neuromuscular:
  - behavioural disturbances
  - hypomania or mania
  - confusional states or delirium (particularly in the elderly)
  - disorientation
  - headache
  - convulsions
  - movement disorders and dyskinesias
  - paraesthesia
  - dysarthria
  - taste disturbance
  - tinnitus
  - EEG changes
  - tremors
- haematological:
  - agranulocytosis
  - leucopenia
  - eosinophilia
  - purpura
  - thrombocytopenia
- allergic:
  - skin rash
  - urticaria
  - photosensitization
  - oedema of the face and tongue
- gastrointestinal:
  - nausea
  - vomiting
  - epigastric distress
  - stomatitis
  - rarely hepatitis (abnormal liver function tests and jaundice)
- endocrine:
  - testicular enlargement and gynaecomastia in males
  - breast enlargement and galactorrhoea in females
  - changes in libido (increased or decreased)
  - impotence
  - blood sugar changes (increased or decreased)
  - syndrome of inappropriate ADH secretion
  - hyponatraemia (which may be caused by inappropriate ADH secretion)

- other:
  - sweating
  - increased appetite
  - weight gain (although weight loss may occur instead)
  - oedema.

Withdrawal symptoms include:
- sudden cessation (after taking the tricyclic antidepressant for a relatively long time)—nausea, headache, and malaise
- gradual cessation—irritability, restlessness, changes in sleep and dreams; these may occur within a fortnight of stopping the tricyclic antidepressant
- rarely, within 1 week of stopping—mania or hypomania.

Caution should be exercised in the following cases:
- cardiovascular disorders
- history of seizures
- impaired liver function
- urinary retention
- narrow-angle glaucoma
- increased intraocular pressure
- hyperthyroidism or patients receiving thyroid medication
- pregnancy
- breastfeeding
- elderly patients
- phaeochromocytoma
- history of mania
- history of psychosis or schizophrenia—psychotic symptoms may be aggravated
- concurrent electroconsulsive therapy
- general anaesthesia—tricyclic antidepressants should be stopped several days before patients undergo elective surgery
- porphyria.

Note also that tricyclic antidepressants augment some of the adverse effects of alcohol.

Contraindications include:
- recent myocardial infarction
- arrhythmias (including heart block)
- mania
- severe liver disease.

Imipramine

℘ Structure

The tricyclic structure of imipramine is shown in Fig. 7.2.

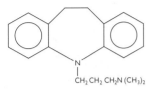

$CH_2\,CH_2\,CH_2N\,(CH_3)_2$

Fig. 7.2 The structure of imipramine.

⚡ Dose

The initial oral adult antidepressant dose is 75mg daily. This can be taken as one dose or it can be divided. According to clinical response, the dose may be raised to between 150–200mg daily (and up to a maximum of 300mg for hospital inpatients); this dose increase should take place gradually, taking care to look out for any evidence of intolerance to the drug. For daily doses of over 150mg, a maximum of 150mg should be given at any one time.

The initial corresponding dose for elderly patients is 10mg daily, very gradually increased, according to clinical response, to between 30–50mg daily.

Imipramine is not recommended for use as an antidepressant in children. (It may, however, be used at doses much lower than adult ones for treating nocturnal enuresis in children.)

☺ Side-effects

See 'Amitriptyline', p.142. Imipramine is less sedating than amitriptyline.

Trimipramine

✀ Structure

The tricyclic structure of trimipramine is shown in Fig. 7.3.

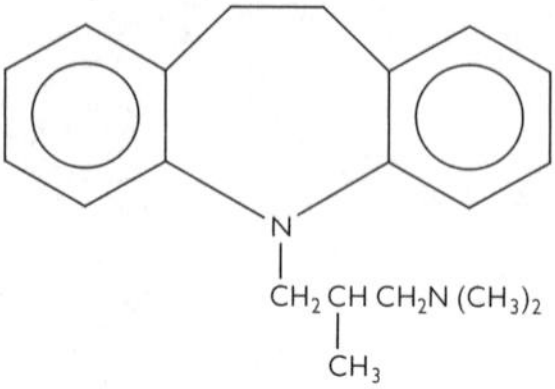

Fig. 7.3 The structure of trimipramine.

⟐ Dose

The initial oral adult antidepressant dose is between 50–75mg daily. This can be taken as one bedtime dose or it can be divided. (Trimipramine is relatively sedating and so can be prescribed to be taken at bedtime in those with insomnia.) According to clinical response, the dose may be raised to between 150–300mg daily; this dose increase should take place gradually, taking care to look out for any evidence of intolerance to the drug.

The initial corresponding dose for elderly patients is between 10–25mg 3 times daily. Half the non-elderly adult dose may be sufficient as a maintenance dose in elderly patients.

Trimipramine is not recommended for use as an antidepressant in children.

☺ Side-effects

See 'Amitriptyline', p.142.

Dosulepin

This tricyclic antidepressant used to be known as dothiepin. As mentioned earlier, dosulepin is particularly dangerous in overdosage and is not recommended for the treatment of depression; it should only be prescribed by a specialist.

Clomipramine

೪ Structure
The tricyclic structure of clomipramine is shown in Fig. 7.4.

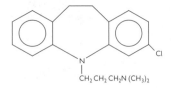

Fig. 7.4 The structure of clomipramine.

ꙮ Dose
The initial oral adult (>18 years) antidepressant dose is 10mg daily. (The initial dose for phobic and obsessional states is 25mg daily.) According to clinical response, the dose may be raised to between 30–150 daily; this dose increase should take place gradually, taking care to look out for any evidence of intolerance to the drug. This maintenance dose may be taken as one bedtime dose or it can be divided. (Clomipramine is relatively sedating and so can be prescribed to be taken at bedtime in those with insomnia.) The maximum recommended *British National Formulary* dose is 250mg daily.

The initial corresponding dose for elderly patients is 10mg daily (for depression, and for phobic and obsessional states). This may be very gradually increased, according to clinical response, over a period no less than 10 days to between 30–75mg daily for depression, taking great care to examine the patient very regularly. (For phobic and obsessional states, the initial dose of 10mg daily in the elderly may be gradually increased, according to clinical response and tolerance, over a fortnight to between 100–150mg daily.)

Clomipramine is not recommended for use as an antidepressant in children.

☺ Side-effects
See 'Amitriptyline', p.142. Clomipramine is also associated with diarrhoea, hypertension, flushing, memory impairment, muscle weakness, myoclonus, muscle hypertonia, fatigue, yawning, and mydriasis.

Lofepramine

𝄇 Structure

The structure of lofepramine is shown in Fig. 7.5.

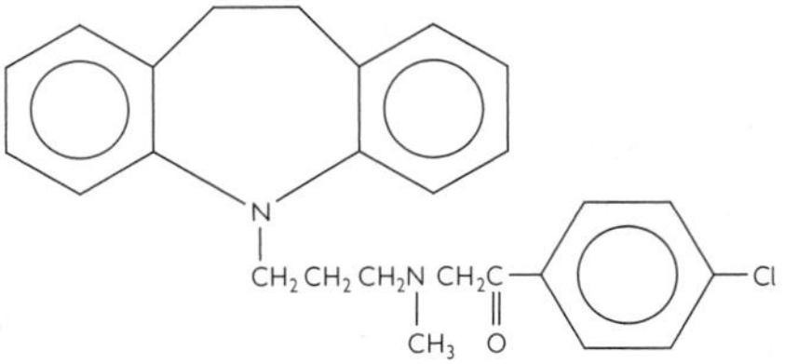

Fig. 7.5 The structure of lofepramine.

𝄏 Dose

The oral adult antidepressant dose is between 140–210mg daily. This should be taken as divided doses; lofepramine is available in 70mg tablets and also as an oral suspension. Elderly patients may respond clinically to a lower dose.

Lofepramine is not recommended for use as an antidepressant in children under the age of 18 years.

☺ Side-effects

See 'Amitriptyline', p.142. Lofepramine is less sedating than amitriptyline, and it is less likely to cause antimuscarinic side-effects and is less likely to be fatal following overdose. On the other hand, lofepramine is more likely than amitriptyline to be associated with liver disorders.

Nortriptyline

⅋ Structure

The tricyclic structure of nortriptyline is shown in Fig. 7.6.

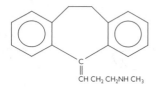

Fig. 7.6 The structure of nortriptyline.

♪ Dose

The oral adult antidepressant maintenance dose is 75–100mg daily (start-ing at a low dose which is gradually raised to this range according to clinical response and tolerability). This can be taken as one dose or it can be divided (typically as 25mg taken 3 or 4 times daily). The maximum recommended dose is 150mg daily.

The oral adult antidepressant maintenance dose for elderly patients is 30–50mg daily, taken in divided doses.

Nortriptyline is not recommended for use as an antidepressant in chil-dren. (It may, however, be used at doses much lower than adult ones for treating nocturnal enuresis in children.)

☺ Side-effects

See 'Amitriptyline', p.142. The manufacturer, King, recommends measur-ing plasma levels of nortriptyline (Allegron®) when the daily dose is above 100mg, with a view to maintaining the nortriptyline plasma level within the optimum range of 50–150ng/mL (that is, 50–150 nanograms per millilitre). Nortriptyline is less sedating than amitriptyline.

Doxepin

❧ Structure

The tricyclic structure of doxepin is shown in Fig. 7.7.

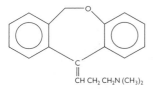

CH CH₂ CH₂N (CH₃)₂

Fig. 7.7 The structure of doxepin.

♪ Dose

The initial oral adult antidepressant dose is 75mg daily. This can be taken as one bedtime dose or it can be divided. (Doxepin is relatively sedating and so can be prescribed to be taken at bedtime in those with insomnia.) According to clinical response, the dose may be raised to 300 daily, taken as 3 divided doses (that is, a maximum of 100mg, 3 times daily); this dose increase should take place gradually, taking care to look out for any evidence of intolerance to the drug. The maximum dose to be taken at any one time is 100mg. The usual maintenance dose is between 30–300mg daily.

The initial corresponding dose for elderly patients is between 10–50mg daily. 30–50mg daily may be sufficient as a maintenance dose in elderly patients.

Doxepin is not recommended for use as an antidepressant in children.

☺ Side-effects

See 'Amitriptyline', p.142.

Trazodone

⅌ Structure

The structure of this tricyclic antidepressant-related antidepressant is shown in Fig. 7.8.

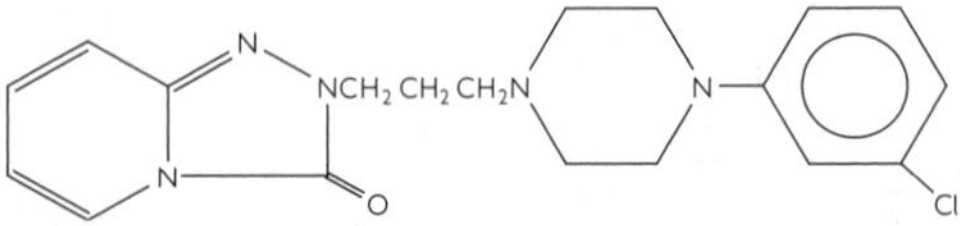

Fig. 7.8 The structure of trazodone.

🗍 Dose

The initial oral adult antidepressant dose is 150mg daily. This can be taken as one bedtime dose or it can be divided (taken after meals). (Trazodone is relatively sedating and so can be prescribed to be taken at bedtime in those with insomnia.) According to clinical response, the dose may be raised to a maximum of 300mg daily; this dose increase should take place gradually, taking care to look out for any evidence of intolerance to the drug. For hospital inpatients the maximum daily dose is 600mg, in divided doses.

The initial corresponding dose for elderly patients is 100mg daily.

Trazodone may also be used as an anxiolytic. The adult dose is 75mg daily, which may be gradually increased to a maximum of 300mg daily.

Trazodone is not recommended for use in children.

☺ Side-effects

See 'Amitriptyline', p.142. Trazodone may cause priapism rarely, when treatment with it should immediately be stopped, but it is less likely than amitriptyline to cause antimuscarinic side-effects or cardiovascular side-effects.

Mianserin

❧ Structure
The structure of this tetracyclic antidepressant is shown in Fig. 7.9.

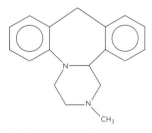

Fig. 7.9 The structure of mianserin.

♪ Dose
The initial oral adult antidepressant dose is 30–40mg daily. This can be taken as one bedtime dose or as divided doses. (Mianserin is relatively sedating and so can be prescribed to be taken at bedtime in those with insomnia.) According to clinical response, the dose may be raised to a maximum of 90mg daily; this dose increase should take place gradually, taking care to look out for any evidence of intolerance to the drug. A full blood count should be carried out every 4 weeks during the first 3 months of pharmacotherapy with mianserin. Clinical signs of blood dyscrasias should be looked for regularly thereafter. The usual adult dose range is between 30–90mg daily.

The initial corresponding dose for elderly patients is 30mg daily. As for non-elderly adult patients, a full blood count should be carried out every 4 weeks during the first 3 months of pharmacotherapy with mianserin. Clinical signs of blood dyscrasias should be looked for regularly thereafter; disorders such as aplastic anaemia are particularly likely to occur in elderly patients treated with mianserin.

Mianserin is not recommended for use in children.

☺ Side-effects
See 'Amitriptyline', p.142. Mianserin may cause leucopenia, agranulocytosis, and aplastic anaemia (particularly in elderly patients). Other side-effects include:
- arthritis
- arthralgia
- jaundice.

Mianserin is less likely than amitriptyline to cause antimuscarinic side-effects or cardiovascular side-effects.

Monoamine-oxidase inhibitors

The use of MAOIs 156
Choice 159
Withdrawal 160
Phenelzine 161
Isocarboxazid 164
Tranylcypromine 165
Reversible MAOIs 166
Moclobemide 167

The use of MAOIs

The enzyme monoamine oxidase (MAO), found mainly in the external mitochondrial membrane, acts on central nervous system neurotransmitters such as noradrenaline, serotonin, and dopamine. The involvement of MAO in the metabolic degradation of noradrenaline is shown in Fig. 8.1. MAO catalyses the catabolism of serotonin into 5-hydroxyindoleacetic acid, or 5-HIAA for short.

Monoamine oxidase inhibitors, conventionally abbreviated to MAOIs, act by inhibiting the metabolic degradation of monoamines by MAO. The differing actions of MAO-A and MAO-B are shown in Fig. 8.2.

Traditional MAOIs are non-selective, inhibiting the actions of both MAO-A and MAO-B (see Fig. 8.3). Since these MAOIs inhibit the peripheral catabolism of pressor amines, and in particular that of dietary tyramine, it is vitally important that patients taking MAOIs avoid foodstuffs that contain tyramine. Eating tyramine-rich food while taking an MAOI can otherwise lead to a potentially fatal hypertensive crisis. Certain drugs, including over-the-counter medicines like cough remedies, should also be avoided while taking MAOIs (see bullet list below). These restrictions have tended to limit the use of MAOIs in non-inpatients.

Foods which must be avoided while being treated with MAOIs include:
- cheese (except cottage cheese and cream cheese)
- meat extracts
- yeast extracts
- fermented soya bean products
- alcohol (particularly chianti, fortified wines and beer)
- non-fresh fish
- non-fresh meat
- non-fresh poultry
- offal
- avocado
- banana skins
- broad-bean pods
- caviar
- herring (pickled or smoked).

Medicines which must be avoided while taking MAOIs include:
- Indirectly-acting sympathomimetic amines, such as:
  - ephedrine
  - fenfluramine.
- Cough mixtures containing sympathomimetics.
- Nasal decongestants containing sympathomimetics.
- L-dopa.
- Opioid analgesics, particularly pethidine.
- Tricyclic antidepressants (the combination of the MAOI tranylcypromine with the tricyclic antidepressant clomipramine is particularly dangerous).

The *British National Formulary* gives the following advice on the use of MAOIs before and after (and indeed in addition to) other antidepressants.

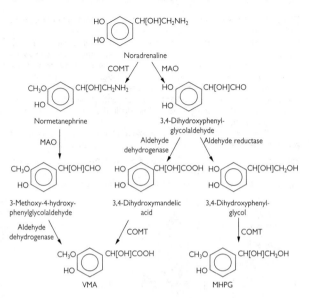

Fig. 8.1 Catabolic pathways for noradrenaline. Reproduced with permission from Puri BK and Tyrer PJ (1998). *Sciences Basic to Psychiatry*, 2nd edn. Churchill Livingstone, Edinburgh.

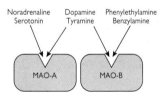

Fig. 8.2 The metabolic degradation of monoamines by MAO-A and MAO-B. Reproduced with permission from Puri BK, Laking PJ, and Treasaden IH (2003). *Textbook of Psychiatry*, 2nd edn. Churchill Livingstone, Edinburgh.

'Other *antidepressants* should **not** be started for 2 weeks after treatment
with MAOIs has been stopped (3 weeks if starting clomipramine or imipramine). Some psychiatrists use selected tricyclics in conjunction with
MAOIs but this is hazardous, indeed potentially lethal, except in experienced hands and there is no evidence that the combination is more
effective than when either constituent is used alone. The combination of
tranylcypromine with clomipramine is particularly **dangerous**.

Conversely, an MAOI should not be started until at least 7–14 days after
a tricyclic or related antidepressant (3 weeks in the case of clomipramine
or imipramine) has been stopped.

In addition, an MAOI should not be started for at least 2 weeks after a
previous MAOI has been stopped (then started at a reduced dose).'

Patients being prescribed MAOIs should be given MAOI treatment cards
which list precautions to be taken. These should be issued to the patient
by either the prescribing doctor or the dispensing pharmacy.

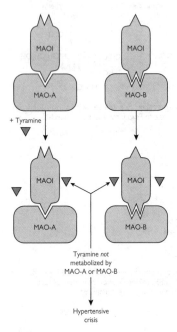

Fig. 8.3 Non-selective and irreversible inhibition of MAO-A and MAO-B by
traditional MAOIs. Reproduced with permission from Puri BK, Laking PJ, and
Treasaden IH (2003). *Textbook of Psychiatry*, 2nd edn. Churchill Livingstone,
Edinburgh.

Choice

Traditional MAOIs which are currently available for prescription fall into two groups:
- Hydrazine:
  - phenelzine
  - isocarboxazid.
- Hon-hydrazine:
  - tranylcypromine.

The non-hydrazine MAOI tranylcypromine may cause dependency. The reason for this is not certain. One possibility put forward is that the cyclopropyl ring of tranylcypromine (see Fig. 8.6) may be cleaved after administration of the drug to form amfetamine (amphetamine), although there is no clear evidence in favour of this possibility (see, for example, Sherry et al., 2000). In contrast, the hydrazine MAOIs, phenelzine, and isocarboxazid, are less likely to be stimulant and cause dependency, and may therefore be preferred clinically to tranylcypromine.

Withdrawal

Withdrawal from pharmacotherapy with MAOIs should ideally take place very gradually.

Phenelzine

ஃ Structure

The structure of this hydrazine MAOI is shown in Fig. 8.4.

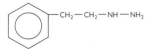

Fig. 8.4 The structure of phenelzine.

✥ Dose

Before starting pharmacotherapy with an MAOI, the patient's blood pressure and liver function tests should be measured; these should be monitored while being treated with the MAOI, which should be discontinued if the patient suffers from palpitations, frequent headaches, or abnormal liver function tests.

The initial oral adult antidepressant dose is 15mg thrice daily (that is, a total of 45mg daily). According to clinical response, after 2 weeks this dose may be raised to 15mg 4 times per day (that is, a total of 60mg daily). The maximum dose for hospitalized inpatients is 90mg daily, taken as 30mg thrice daily. The dose of phenelzine should then be reduced gradually to the minimum effective maintenance dose, which may be 15mg every other day (that is, the equivalent of 7.5mg daily).

Elderly patients are particularly susceptible to the side-effect of postural hypotension, and in general it is better not to prescribe an MAOI for them. If an MAOI is to be used, great caution should be exercised, and it is prudent to start on a lower initial dose of 15mg daily (preferably given in the morning).

Phenelzine is not recommended for use in children.

☺ Side-effects

Common side-effects of phenelzine include:
- postural hypotension
- dizziness
- light-headedness.

Less common side-effects include:
- blurred vision
- drowsiness
- insomnia
- agitation
- weakness
- fatigue
- dry mouth
- diarrhoea or constipation
- fast pounding heartbeat
- peripheral oedema—particularly of the feet and/or lower legs

- myoclonic movements
- tremors
- muscle twitching during sleep
- hyperreflexia
- euphoria, unusual excitement or nervousness
- cardiac arrhythmias
- nystagmus
- micturition difficulties
- increased sweating
- convulsions
- rashes
- purpura
- sexual function side-effects, including reduced libido
- weight gain
- increased appetite—particularly for sweets
- leucopenia
- nausea
- raised liver enzymes.

Rare side-effects include:
- dark urine
- pyrexia
- slurred speech
- sore throat
- jaundice
- fatal progressive hepatocellular necrosis
- decreased appetite
- paraesthesia
- peripheral neuritis
- peripheral neuropathy.

Psychosis may be precipitated in those who are susceptible.
  Caution should be exercised in the following cases:
- diabetes mellitus
- cardiovascular disease
- concurrent electroconvulsive therapy
- epilepsy
- blood disorders
- elderly patients
- porphyria
- pregnancy
- breast-feeding
- surgery—MAOIs should be stopped at least 2 weeks before (elective) surgery.

Contraindications include:
- phaeochromocytoma
- hepatic impairment
- abnormal liver function tests
- cerebrovascular disease

- congestive cardiac failure
- mania.

Note the dangerous potential food and medication interactions mentioned earlier in this chapter. Taking these with an MAOI can lead to:
- hypertensive crisis
- convulsive seizures
- pyrexia
- marked sweating
- excitation
- delirium
- tremor
- coma
- circulatory collapse
- death.

Isocarboxazid

❧ Structure

The structure of this hydrazine MAOI is shown in Fig. 8.5.

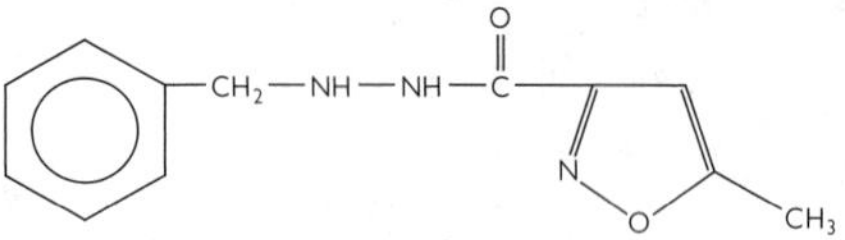

Fig. 8.5 The structure of isocarboxazid.

♣ Dose

Before starting pharmacotherapy with an MAOI, the patient's blood pressure and liver function tests should be measured; these should be monitored while being treated with the MAOI, which should be discontinued if the patient suffers from palpitations, frequent headaches, or abnormal liver function tests.

The initial oral adult antidepressant dose of isocarboxazid is 30mg daily (either as a single dose or taken in divided doses). According to clinical response, after 4 weeks this dose may be raised to a maximum of 60mg per day for 4–6 weeks, while carefully monitoring the patient (preferably as an inpatient). The dose of isocarboxazid should then be reduced gradually to the minimum effective maintenance dose, which is usually between 10–20mg daily, but might be as high as 40mg daily.

Elderly patients are particularly susceptible to the side-effect of postural hypotension, and in general it is better not to prescribe an MAOI for them. If isocarboxazid is to be used, the total dose given should be no more than 5–10mg daily.

Isocarboxazid is not recommended for use in children.

☻ Side-effects

As listed for phenelzine and MAOIs in general.

Tranylcypromine

✤ Structure

This is a non-hydrazine MAOI. Its structure is shown in Fig. 8.6.

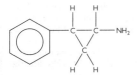

Fig. 8.6 The structure of tranylcypromine.

♣ Dose

Before starting pharmacotherapy with an MAOI, the patient's blood pressure and liver function tests should be measured; these should be monitored while being treated with the MAOI, which should be discontinued if the patient suffers from palpitations, frequent headaches, or abnormal liver function tests.

The initial oral adult antidepressant dose of tranylcypromine is 20mg daily. This should be administered as 10mg twice daily, with the second dose being given no later than three in the afternoon. This is to avoid causing insomnia (which can occur if tranylcypromine, being a stimulating antidepressant, is taken in the evening). According to the clinical response, after 1 week this dose may be raised to 30mg per day, given as 10mg in the morning and 20mg no later than three in the afternoon. (Doses above 30mg daily should only be used exceptionally, in closely monitored patients.) The dose of tranylcypromine should then be reduced gradually to the minimum effective maintenance dose, which is usually 10mg daily.

Elderly patients are particularly susceptible to the side-effect of postural hypotension, and in general it is better not to prescribe an MAOI for them.

Tranylcypromine is not recommended for use in children.

☺ Side-effects

As listed for phenelzine and MAOIs in general. Note that tranylcypromine is more likely than other MAOIs to cause a hypertensive crisis with a throbbing headache (when the drug should be discontinued).

In addition to those noted under phenelzine, an added contraindication in the case of tranylcypromine is hyperthyroidism.

Reversible MAOIs

Reversible MAOIs (or RIMAs for short) selectively and reversibly inhibit just MAO-A. Therefore they preferentially reduce the catabolism of the monoamines noradrenaline and serotonin (see Fig. 8.2, p.157) by MAO-A. As the binding is reversible, RIMAs can be displaced by substances such as tyramine, as shown in Fig. 8.7. Therefore, RIMAs are much less likely to cause a food or drug interaction leading to a hypertensive crisis. (In contrast, conventional MAOIs are irreversible inhibitors of MAO-A and MAO-B.)

The first RIMA to be introduced into clinical practice was moclobemide. In addition to be used as an antidepressant, moclobemide is also licensed for the treatment of social anxiety disorder (social phobia).

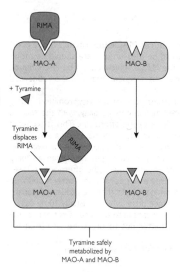

Fig. 8.7 Selective and reversible inhibition of MAO-A by RIMAs. Reproduced with permission from Puri BK, Laking PJ, and Treasaden IH (2003). *Textbook of Psychiatry*, 2nd edn. Churchill Livingstone, Edinburgh.

Moclobemide

℘ Structure

The structure of moclobemide is shown in Fig. 8.8.

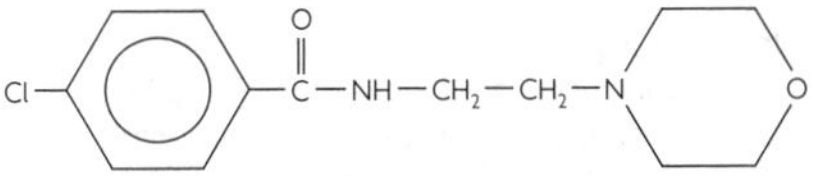

Cl—⟨benzene ring⟩—C(=O)—NH—CH$_2$—CH$_2$—N⟨morpholine ring with O⟩

Fig. 8.8 The structure of moclobemide.

∴ Dose

The initial oral adult antidepressant dose is 300mg daily, which is usu-ally administered in divided doses taken after meals. According to clin-ical response, this dose may be altered to a usual therapeutic range of between 150–600mg daily (with doses of 300mg or more daily being taken as divided doses after meals).

For social anxiety disorder, the initial adult dose of moclobemide is also 300mg daily, which is doubled on day four to 300mg twice daily (that is, a total dose of 600mg daily). The clinical efficacy of this higher dose is then assessed over the next 8–12 weeks.

Moclobemide is not recommended for use in children (as either a treat-ment for depression or for social anxiety disorder).

☺ Side-effects

Relatively common side-effects of moclobemide include:

- sleep disturbances
- agitation
- restlessness
- feelings of anxiety
- dizziness
- headache
- paraesthesia
- dry mouth
- visual disturbances
- gastrointestinal disorders
- dermatological reactions—e.g. rash, pruritus, flushing, urticaria
- oedema.

Rare side-effects include:

- confusional states—these resolve rapidly on discontinuation of the moclobemide
- raised liver enzymes (without clinical sequelae)
- galactorrhoea
- hyponatraemia.

Although RIMAs are much safer than traditional MAOIs, being less likely to lead to a hypertensive crisis when a patient on a RIMA eats tyramine-

containing food or takes a sympathomimetic medication, it is prudent for patients taking moclobemide to:
- avoid ingesting large quantities of tyramine-rich food
- avoid sympathomimetic medication (e.g. ephedrine and pseudoephedrine).

Moclobemide should not be prescribed with selegiline or pethidine or with another antidepressant drug; this is particularly true of the tricyclic antidepressant clomipramine. The elimination half-life at a dose of 300mg twice daily is only around 3 hours, and so it is safe to switch from moclobemide to another antidepressant without needing a treatment-free period. However, if switching from another antidepressant to moclobemide, a treatment-free period is needed, as follows:
- At least 5 weeks if switching from fluoxetine.
- At least 2 weeks if switching from sertraline.
- At least 1 week if switching from another SSRI (other than fluoxetine or sertraline) or from a tricyclic antidepressant, tricyclic-related antidepressant or MAOI.

Caution should be exercised in the following cases:
- agitation
- excited patients
- thyrotoxicosis (theoretical risk of a hypertensive crisis)
- hepatic impairment
- bipolar disorder—a risk of manic relapse
- pregnancy
- breastfeeding.

Contraindications include:
- acute confusional state
- phaeochromocytoma—a theoretical risk of a hypertensive crisis.

Selective serotonin re-uptake inhibitors

The use of SSRIs 170
Risk of suicide or hostility 171
Interactions with MAOIs 172
Withdrawal reactions and dependency 173
Side-effects of SSRIs 174
Efficacy 176
Fluvoxamine 177
Fluoxetine 178
Sertraline 180
Paroxetine 182
Citalopram 184
Escitalopram 186

The use of SSRIs

As implied by their name, the selective serotonin re-uptake inhibitors, commonly abbreviated to SSRIs, selectively inhibit the re-uptake of the neurotransmitter serotonin (also known as 5-hydroxytryptamine or 5-HT for short). The major SSRIs in clinical use are:

- fluvoxamine (which was the first SSRI to be introduced into clinical practice in the UK, in 1987)
- fluoxetine (launched in the UK in 1989)
- sertraline (launched in the UK in 1990)
- paroxetine (launched in the UK in 1991)
- citalopram (launched in the UK in 1995)
- escitalopram (launched in the UK in 2002).

In contrast to tricyclic antidepressants, tricyclic-like antidepressants and MAOIs (see Chapters 7 and 8), SSRIs and SSRI-related antidepressants (see Chapter 10) were promoted as having the virtue of being safer in overdose and, unlike tricyclic antidepressants, being less likely to cause antimuscarinic and cardiac side-effects.

Risk of suicide or hostility

Starting in the 1990s, the use of SSRIs has become increasingly controversial. In particular, it has been suggested that there appears to be a risk of suicidal and perhaps even homicidal thoughts in patients who receive SSRI medication; this risk appears to be increased when there is a change in dosage of the SSRI (either an increase—including starting the drug in the first place—or a decrease). For example, the review by Healy and Whitaker (2003) of randomized controlled trials, meta-analyses of clinical trials, and epidemiological studies undertaken to investigate this issue concluded that

'These same [randomized controlled trials]…revealed an excess of suicidal acts on active treatments compared with placebo, with an odds ratio of 2.4 (95% confidence interval 1.6–3.7). This excess of suicidal acts also appears in epidemiological studies. The data reviewed here make it difficult to sustain a null hypothesis that SSRIs do not cause problems in some individuals.'

On the other hand, there have been several systematic studies which have failed to detect such a risk in adults (Isacsson et al., 2005; Gibbons et al., 2005; Martinez et al., 2005; Fazel et al., 2006), although there is some evidence of a possible risk in those aged 18 years or younger, particularly if unpublished trial results are taken into account (see, for example, Whittington et al., 2004; Martinez et al., 2005). The issue remains controversial (see, for example, Goldsmith and Moncrieff, 2011).

The *British National Formulary* (62nd edition; September 2011) gives the following advice:

'Depressive illness in children and adolescents

The balance of risks and benefits for the treatment of depressive illness in individuals under 18 years is considered unfavourable for the SSRIs citalopram, escitalopram, paroxetine, and sertraline, and for mirtazapine and venlafaxine. Clinical trials have failed to show efficacy and have shown an increase in harmful outcomes. However, it is recognised that specialists may sometimes decide to use these drugs in response to individual clinical need; children and adolescents should be monitored carefully for suicidal behaviour, self-harm or hostility, particularly at the beginning of treatment.

Only fluoxetine has been shown in clinical trials to be effective for treating depressive illness in children and adolescents. However, it is possible that, in common with the other SSRIs, it is associated with a small risk of self-harm and suicidal thoughts. Overall, the balance of risks and benefits for fluoxetine in the treatment of depressive illness in individuals under 18 years is considered favourable, but children and adolescents must be carefully monitored as above.'

All patients being treated with SSRIs and SSRI-like antidepressants should be regularly checked for evidence of:

- hostility
- self-harm
- suicidal behaviour.

This is particularly important at the time of sudden changes in dosage, including:

- at the start of treatment
- at the time of dose change (in either direction).

Interactions with MAOIs

Treatment with an MAOI should be stopped at least 2 weeks before starting treatment with an SSRI or related antidepressant. However, if switching from an SSRI to an MAOI (or to the RIMA moclobemide), a treatment-free period is needed, as follows:

- at least 5 weeks if switching from fluoxetine
- at least 2 weeks if switching from sertraline
- at least 1 week if switching from another SSRI (other than fluoxetine or sertraline).

Withdrawal reactions and dependency

The following advice has been issued by the Committee on Safety of Medicines (CSM) (from the *Report of the CSM Expert Working Group on the Safety of Selective Serotonin Reuptake Inhibitor Antidepressants*, December 2004):

'It has been known for some time that, as with other antidepressants, the SSRIs and related antidepressants are associated with withdrawal reactions, although different SSRIs appear to cause withdrawal reactions to different extents. The Group considered data from clinical trials, the published literature and spontaneous reports from health professionals and patients. The Group's conclusions can be summarized as follows:

- All SSRIs may be associated with withdrawal reactions on stopping or reducing treatment. Paroxetine and venlafaxine seem to be associated with a greater frequency of withdrawal reactions than other SSRIs. [Paroxetine and venlafaxine have relatively short half-lives.] A proportion of SSRI withdrawal reactions are severe and disabling to the individual.
- The most commonly experienced withdrawal reactions are dizziness, numbness and tingling, gastrointestinal disturbances (particularly nausea and vomiting), headache, sweating, anxiety and sleep disturbances.
- Awareness of the risk of withdrawal reactions associated with SSRIs needs to be increased amongst both prescribers and patients.
- There is evidence that withdrawal reactions are less severe when the dose is tapered gradually over a period of several weeks, according to the patient's need. Availability of low dose formulations to allow gradual titration is important.
- There is no clear evidence that the SSRIs and related antidepressants have a significant dependence liability or show development of a dependence syndrome according to internationally accepted criteria (either DSM-IV or ICD-10).'

Side-effects of SSRIs

The following side-effects apply to all the SSRIs. Additional side-effects that relate to individual SSRIs are listed for each drug.

- general:
  - hypersensitivity reaction—may include rash and vasculitis; it is probably prudent to stop the SSRI if an otherwise unexplained skin rash appears
  - urticaria
  - angio-oedema
  - anaphylactoid reaction
  - asthenia
  - chills
  - dry mouth
  - photosensitivity
  - pruritus
  - serum sickness-like reaction
  - sweating
  - vasodilatation
  - arthralgia
  - myalgia
  - hyponatraemia (may be caused by inappropriate ADH secretion)
  - galactorrhoea
- gastrointestinal:
  - nausea
  - vomiting
  - dyspepsia
  - abdominal pain
  - diarrhoea
  - constipation
  - dysphagia
  - taste alteration
- haematological:
  - ecchymosis
  - purpura
- nervous system:
  - hypomania or mania
  - anxiety
  - headache
  - insomnia
  - tremor
  - dizziness
  - asthenia
  - hallucinations
  - drowsiness
  - convulsions
  - movement disorders and dyskinesias
  - blurred vision
  - mydriasis
  - impaired concentration

- urogenital:
  - anorgasmia
  - delayed or absent ejaculation
  - priapism
  - prolonged penile erection
  - impotence
  - reduced libido
  - urinary frequency
  - urinary retention.

Caution should be exercised in the following cases:
- epilepsy or a history of seizures
- if receiving electroconvulsive therapy—there have been reports of prolonged seizures in patients taking fluoxetine
- a history of hypomania or mania—(hypo)mania may be induced by an SSRI
- cardiac disease
- diabetes mellitus—hypoglycaemia may occur during SSRI treatment, an hyperglycaemia may develop following SSRI discontinuation; insulin and/or oral hypoglycaemic drug doses may need to be changed when SSRI treatment is initiated or discontinued
- susceptibility to angle-closure glaucoma
- patients being treated with drugs which increase the bleeding time (e.g. warfarin)
- history of bleeding disorders
- hepatic impairment
- renal impairment
- pregnancy
- breastfeeding
- patients being treated with diuretics—such patients, particularly if elderly, may develop hyponatraemia while taking an SSRI.

The performance of skilled tasks such as operating machinery or driving may be impaired by SSRI pharmacotherapy.

As already mentioned, withdrawal of SSRI treatment should take place very gradually.

SSRIs are contraindicated in hypomania or mania.

Efficacy

It has been suggested that SSRIs may not, in fact, be efficacious in treating depressive illness. For example, Professor Irving Kirsch reviewed meta-analyses in which response to SSRIs and to placebo were calculated (Kirsch, 2009), and reported that:

'All but one of these meta-analyses included unpublished as well as published trials. Most trials failed to show a significant advantage of SSRIs over inert placebo, and the differences between drug and placebo are not clinically significant for most depressed patients. Documents obtained from the U.S. Food and Drug Administration (FDA) revealed an explicit decision to keep this information from the public and from prescribing physicians.'

Fluvoxamine

℘ Structure
The structure of this fluorinated SSRI is shown in Fig. 9.1.

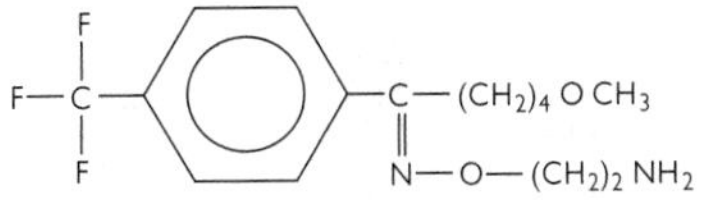

Fig. 9.1 The structure of fluvoxamine.

⚕ Dose
The initial oral adult (>18 years) antidepressant dose is 50–100mg daily, which is usually administered in the evening. According to clinical response, this dose may be gradually increased to a maximum of 300mg daily (with doses of 150mg or more daily being taken as divided doses). The mainte-nance dose is usually 100mg daily.

The initial oral adult dose for obsessive–compulsive disorder is 50mg each evening. According to clinical response, this dose may be gradually increased to a maximum of 300mg daily (with doses of 150mg or more daily being taken as divided doses). The maintenance dose for obsessive–compulsive disorder is usually between 100–300mg daily. For children over the age of 8 years, the initial dose for obsessive–compulsive disorder is 25mg daily. This may be increased, according to clinical response, in increments of 25mg every 4–7 days, to a maximum of 200mg daily (with doses of 50mg or more daily being taken as divided doses). Treatment with fluvoxamine for obsessive–compulsive disorder should be reconsid-ered if there is no improvement in symptomatology within 10 weeks.

☺ Side-effects
See 'Side-effects of SSRIs', p.174. In addition, fluvoxamine may cause:
• palpitations
• tachycardia
• malaise.

More rarely, fluvoxamine may also cause:
• postural hypotension
• confusional states
• ataxia.

In addition to the cautions listed in 'Side-effects of SSRIs', note that it is also best to avoid concomitant use of this SSRI with either theophylline or aminophylline.

Fluoxetine

℀ Structure

The structure of this fluorinated SSRI, which has a very long half-life, is shown in Fig. 9.2.

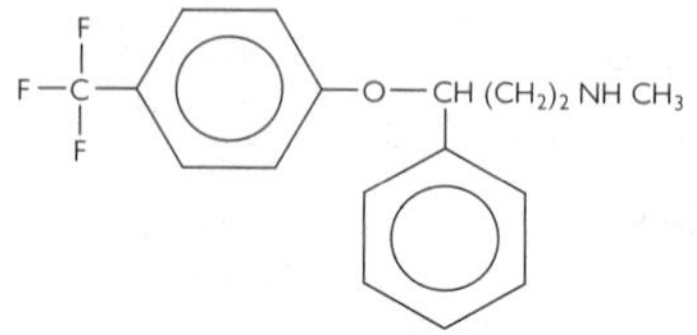

Fig. 9.2 The structure of fluoxetine.

♪ Dose

The initial oral adult antidepressant dose is 20mg daily, which is usually administered in the morning. According to clinical response, after 3–4weeks this dose may be gradually increased to a maximum of 60mg (40mg being the usual maximum for the elderly) daily.

For children aged between 8–18 years, the initial dose of fluoxetine is 10mg daily, which may be increased if need be, according to clinical response, after 1–2 weeks, to a maximum of 20mg daily. (However, see the comments earlier in this chapter about the use of SSRIs in children and adolescents—' Risk of suicide or hostility', p.171.)

The initial oral adult (>18 years) dose for *obsessive–compulsive disorder* is 20mg daily, which is usually administered in the morning. According to clinical response, after 2 weeks this dose may be gradually increased to a maximum of 60mg (usually a maximum of 40mg for the elderly) daily. The maintenance dose is usually 20–60mg (20–40mg for the elderly) daily. Treatment with fluoxetine for obsessive–compulsive disorder should be reconsidered if there is no improvement in symptomatology within 10 weeks.

The initial oral adult (>18 years) dose for *bulimia nervosa* is 60mg daily (taken either as one dose, usually in the morning, or as a divided dose).

☺ Side-effects

See 'Side-effects of SSRIs', p.174. In addition, fluoxetine may cause:
- alopecia
- blood glucose changes
- chills
- confusion
- dyspnoea
- euphoria
- impairment of concentration
- pharyngitis

- postural hypotension
- sleep disturbance
- taste disturbance
- urinary frequency
- vasodilatation
- yawning.

More rarely, fluoxetine may also be associated with pulmonary inflammation and fibrosis. Very rarely, fluoxetine treatment may be associated with a neuroleptic malignant syndrome-like phenomenon.

Sertraline

ஃ Structure

The structure of this chlorinated SSRI is shown in Fig. 9.3.

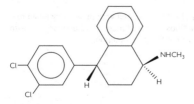

Fig. 9.3 The structure of sertraline.

⁙ Dose

The initial oral adult (>18 years) antidepressant dose is 50mg daily. According to clinical response, over several weeks this dose may be gradually increased, by steps of 50mg, to a maximum of 200mg daily. The maintenance dose is usually 50mg daily.

The initial oral dose for *obsessive–compulsive disorder* is 50mg daily for adults and for adolescents over the age of 12 years. According to clinical response, over several weeks this dose may be gradually increased, by steps of 50mg (over an interval of at least 1 week between increments), to a maximum of 200mg daily. The maintenance dose is usually 50–200mg daily. For children aged between 6–12 years, the initial oral dose for obsessive–compulsive disorder is 25mg daily, increased to 50mg daily after 1 week; according to clinical response, this may be increased in steps of 50mg at intervals of at least 1 week to a maximum of 200mg daily.

The initial oral adult (>18 years) dose for *panic disorder, post-traumatic stress disorder*, or *social anxiety disorder* (social phobia) is 25mg daily, increased after 1 week to 50mg daily. According to clinical response, if this SSRI is well-tolerated and there is partial symptomatic response, over several weeks this dose may be gradually increased, by steps of 50mg (over an interval of at least 1 week between increments), to a maximum of 200mg daily.

☺ Side-effects

See 'Side-effects of SSRIs', p.174. In addition, sertraline treatment may be associated with:

- confusional states
- amnesia
- aggressive behaviour
- pancreatitis
- hepatitis
- jaundice
- hepatic failure

- bronchospasm
- paraesthesia
- stomatitis
- palpitations
- hypertension
- hypercholesterolaemia
- tachycardia
- postural hypotension
- tinnitus
- hypoglycaemia
- leucopenia
- hypothyroidism
- hyperprolactinaemia
- menstrual irregularities
- urinary incontinence.

Paroxetine

✤ Structure

The structure of this chlorinated SSRI is shown in Fig. 9.4.

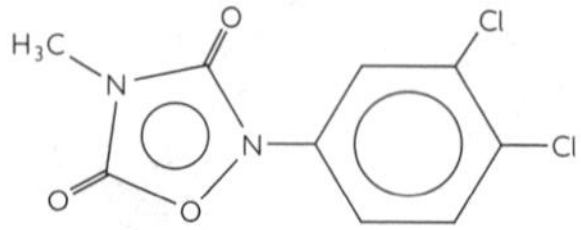

Fig. 9.4 The structure of paroxetine.

♫ Dose

The initial oral adult (>18 years) dose for *depression, social anxiety disorder, post-traumatic stress disorder*, and *generalized anxiety* disorder is 20mg daily, which is usually administered in the morning. According to clinical response, this dose may be gradually increased, in steps of 10mg, to a maximum of 50mg (40mg for the elderly) daily. The CSM recommend that the initial dose of 20mg is sufficient and need not be increased when using paroxetine to treat depression, social anxiety disorder, post-traumatic stress disorder, or generalized anxiety disorder.

The initial oral adult (>18 years) dose for *obsessive–compulsive disorder* is 20mg daily, which is usually administered in the morning. According to clinical response, this dose may be gradually increased, in steps of 10mg, to a maximum of 60mg (40mg for the elderly) daily, with a usual maintenance dose of 40mg daily. The CSM recommend that a dose of 40mg is sufficient and need not be increased further when using paroxetine to treat obsessive–compulsive disorder.

The initial oral adult (>18 years) dose for *panic disorder* is 10mg daily, which is usually administered in the morning. This dose is gradually increased, in steps of 10mg, to a maximum of 60mg (40mg for the elderly) daily, with a usual maintenance dose of 40mg daily. The CSM recommend that a dose of 40mg is sufficient and need not be increased further when using paroxetine to treat panic disorder.

☹ Side-effects

See 'Side-effects of SSRIs', p.174. In addition, paroxetine may cause:
• yawning
• abnormal dreams
• raised cholesterol
• cardiac arrhythmia
• urinary incontinence
• confusional states.

Rarely, paroxetine may cause:
- panic attacks and increased anxiety—indeed, in the initial phase of treatment of panic disorder with this SSRI, panic symptoms may be worsened
- a neuroleptic malignant syndrome-like phenomenon
- depersonalization
- restless legs syndrome.

Paroxetine may be more likely than the other SSRIs to cause a withdrawal syndrome (see 'Withdrawal reactions and dependency', p.174) and to cause extrapyramidal side-effects including orofacial dystonias.

Citalopram

℞ Structure

The structure of this fluorinated SSRI is shown in Fig. 9.5.

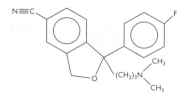

Fig. 9.5 The structure of citalopram.

⚗ Dose

The initial adult oral antidepressant dose is 20mg daily, taken as one dose. According to clinical response, this dose may be gradually increased (in increments of 20mg daily with 3–4 weeks between increments) to a maximum of 40mg (20mg in the elderly aged over 65 years and those with reduced hepatic function) daily.

The initial adult (>18 years) oral dose for *panic disorder* is 10mg daily gradually increased in increments of 10mg daily to the usual maintenance dose of 20–30mg daily. This dose may be gradually increased to a maximum of 40mg (20mg in the elderly aged >65 years and those with reduced hepatic function) daily.

☹ Side-effects

See 'Side-effects of SSRIs', p.174. Citalopram is associated with dose-dependent QT interval prolongation. In view of this, the manufacturer recommends the following.

• Citalopram is contraindicated in patients with known QT interval prolongation or congenital long QT syndrome.
• Use of citalopram with other medicines known to prolong the QT interval is contraindicated.
• Caution is advised in patients at higher risk of developing torsade de pointes, for example, those with congestive cardiac failure, recent myocardial infarction, bradyarrhythmias, or a predisposition to hypokalaemia or hypomagnesaemia because of concomitant illness or medicines.
• Patients should be advised to contact a healthcare professional immediately if they experience an abnormal heart rate or rhythm while taking citalopram.

In addition, citalopram may cause:
• hepatitis
• tachycardia
• palpitations
• bradycardia

- postural hypotension
- coughing
- yawning
- rhinitis
- tinnitus
- confusional states
- malaise
- abnormal dreams
- migraine
- paraesthesia
- taste disturbance
- hypersalivation
- poor concentration
- amnesia
- behavioural disturbance
- euphoria
- mydriasis
- micturition disorders and polyuria
- oedema.

There may be a paradoxical increase in anxiety in the first phase of the treatment of panic disorder with this drug; if this occurs, the dose of citalopram should be reduced.

Escitalopram

⚬ Structure

Escitalopram is the active (S) isomer of citalopram. Therefore, in theory it should be possible to obtain the same benefits as with citalopram, but by using only half the dose of the latter. This should mean that side-effects are less common than with citalopram.

⚬ Dose

The initial adult (aged between 18–65 years) oral antidepressant dose is 10mg daily, taken as one dose. According to clinical response, this dose may be increased to a maximum of 20mg daily. In elderly patients (>65 years), the initial oral antidepressant dose is 5mg daily; the maximum dose of escitalopram for the elderly is 10mg daily.

The initial adult (aged between 18–65 years) oral dose for panic disorder is 5mg daily increased after 1 week to 10mg daily. This dose may be gradually increased to a maximum of 20mg. In elderly patients (>65 years), the initial oral dose for panic disorder is 2.5mg daily, and a lower maintenance dose may suffice; the maximum dose of escitalopram for the elderly is 10mg daily.

The initial adult (aged between 18–65 years) oral dose for social anxiety disorder is 10mg daily. This may be altered after 2–4 weeks according to clinical response. The usual dose is between 5–20mg daily.

☺ Side-effects

See 'Side-effects of SSRIs', p.174. Escitalopram is associated with dose-dependent QT interval prolongation. In view of this, the manufacturer recommends the following:

- Escitalopram is contraindicated in patients with known QT interval prolongation or congenital long QT syndrome.
- Use of escitalopram with other medicines known to prolong the QT interval is contraindicated.
- Caution is advised in patients at higher risk of developing torsade de pointes, for example, those with uncompensated cardiac failure, recent myocardial infarction, bradyarrhythmias, or a predisposition to hypokalaemia or hypomagnesaemia because of concomitant illness or medicines.
- Patients should be advised to contact a healthcare professional immediately if they experience an abnormal heart rate or rhythm while taking escitalopram.

In addition, escitalopram may cause:

- yawning
- sinusitis
- fatigue
- restlessness
- abnormal dreams
- paraesthesia
- pyrexia
- taste disturbance

- bruxism
- oedema
- a confusional state
- syncope
- tachycardia
- epistaxis
- mydriasis
- tinnitus
- alopecia
- menstrual disturbances
- pruritus.

Other and newer antidepressants

Agomelatine *190*
Duloxetine *192*
Flupentixol *195*
Mirtazapine *196*
Reboxetine *198*
Venlafaxine *200*
Tryptophan *204*

Agomelatine

Agomelatine is a new antidepressant with MT_1 and MT_2 melatonergic agonist and $5\text{-}HT_{2C}$ antagonist actions which has been shown to be effective in severe depression (see Mongomery and Kasper, 2007). These properties, together with its lack of major effects on the uptake of dopamine, serotonin, and noradrenaline, may account for its relative lack of adverse side-effects. As Sansone and Sansone (2011) have commented regarding agomelatine:

'The melatonergic function appears to improve sleep patterns, whereas the serotonergic antagonism results in the release of norepinephrine [noradrenaline] and dopamine. Given the current information, the overall side-effect profile of agomelatine appears relatively mild. For example, agomelatine has no discontinuation syndrome, exhibits infrequent sexual dysfunction, and is generally weight neutral. The drug appears to be relatively safe in overdose.'

❧ Structure

The structure of agomelatine is shown in Fig. 10.1.

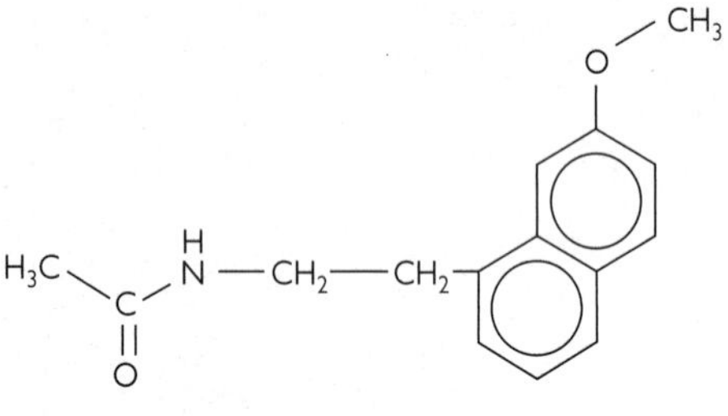

Fig. 10.1 The structure of agomelatine.

♪ Dose

The initial adult (>18 years) oral antidepressant dose is 25mg nocte. This can be increased, according to clinical response, to 50mg nocte after 2 weeks. Liver function tests should be carried out prior to treatment and then at the 6-, 12-, and 24-week time-points, and then as appropriate. If the serum transaminase is higher than 3× the reference range upper limit, then treatment with agomelatine should be stopped.

☻ Side-effects

The commonest side-effects are:
- nausea
- diarrhoea
- constipation
- abdominal pain
- increased serum transaminases
- headache

- dizziness
- drowsiness
- insomnia
- fatigue
- anxiety
- back pain
- sweating.

Less common side-effects include:
- paraesthesia
- eczema
- blurred vision.

Caution should be exercised in the following cases:
- elderly patients
- (hypo)mania
- concomitant use of drugs associated with hepatic injury
- excessive intake of alcohol.

Contraindications include:
- dementia
- hepatic impairment
- breastfeeding.

Duloxetine

This drug inhibits the central re-uptake of serotonin and noradrenaline (norepinephrine).

℞ Structure

The structure of duloxetine is shown in Fig. 10.2.

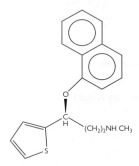

Fig. 10.2 The structure of duloxetine.

♪ Dose

The adult (>18 years) oral antidepressant dose is 60mg once daily.

For the treatment of generalized anxiety disorder, the initial adult (>18 years) dose is 30mg daily, which may be increased as clinically appropriate to 60mg once daily. The maximum dose is 120mg daily.

☺ Side-effects

The commonest side-effects are:
- nausea
- vomiting
- dyspepsia
- constipation
- diarrhoea
- abdominal pain
- flatulence
- dry mouth
- hot flushes
- decreased appetite
- weight change
- palpitations
- abnormal dreams
- paraesthesia
- sweating
- fatigue
- increased sweating

- anxiety
- dizziness
- headache
- tremor
- nervousness
- anorexia
- blurred vision
- sexual dysfunction
- thirst
- lethargy
- drowsiness
- weakness
- pruritus.

Less common side-effects include:
- halitosis
- bruxism
- gastritis
- hepatitis
- tachycardia
- hypertension
- postural hypotension
- syncope
- vertigo
- increased cholesterol
- cold extremities
- disturbance of taste sensation
- impairment of temperature regulation
- poor attention
- movement disorders
- musculoskeletal pain
- twitching
- stomatitis
- thirst
- photosensitivity
- hypothyroidism
- urinary disorders.

It may very rarely be associated with hyponatraemia.
Caution should be exercised in the following cases:
- elderly patients
- cardiac disease
- hypertension
- history of (hypo)mania
- history of seizures
- raised intraocular pressure
- bleeding disorders
- concomitant pharmacotherapy with agents which increase the bleeding time.

Contraindications include:
- hepatic impairment
- renal impairment (if estimated glomerular filtration rate (eGFR) <30mL/min/1.73 m^2)
- pregnancy
- breastfeeding
- narrow-angle glaucoma—duloxetine may be associated with increased mydriasis in patients with uncontrolled narrow-angle glaucoma.

This antidepressant should only be withdrawn gradually.

Flupentixol

This antipsychotic drug has been considered in Chapter 3 (p.66). It can also be used as an antidepressant.

℅ Structure

This is shown in Fig. 3.7 (p.66).

♣ Dose

The initial antidepressant adult (>18 years) dose is 1mg (500 micrograms in the elderly) each morning, increased if needed, according to clinical response, after 1 week to 2mg (1mg in the elderly). The maximum dose is 3mg (1.5mg for the elderly) daily; doses greater than 2mg (1mg in the elderly) daily should be divided, with the last dose being taken no later than four in the afternoon. If there is no beneficial clinical response after 1 week of pharmacotherapy at the maximum dose, then the flupentixol should be discontinued.

☺ Side-effects

See Chapter 3 (p.66).

Mirtazapine

This antidepressant is a presynaptic α_2-antagonist which increases central neurotransmission by noradrenaline (norepinephrine) and serotonin. It was introduced into the UK in 1997. A recent Cochrane review comparing mirtazapine with other antidepressants (Watanabe et al., 2011) found that:

- There was no robust evidence to detect a difference between mirtazapine and tricyclic antidepressants in terms of the response outcome at 2 weeks and at end of the acute-phase treatment (at 6–12 weeks).
- In comparison with SSRIs, mirtazapine was significantly more effective in terms of response at 2 weeks and at the end of acute-phase treatment.
- Mirtazapine was significantly more effective than venlafaxine at 2 weeks and at the end of the acute-phase treatment.
- There was no robust evidence to detect a difference between mirtazapine and trazodone at 2 weeks or at the end of the acute-phase treatment.
- There was no robust evidence to detect a difference between mirtazapine and reboxetine in terms of the response outcome at 2 weeks and at end of the acute-phase treatment.

Structure

The structure of mirtazapine is shown in Fig. 10.3.

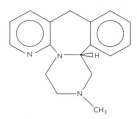

Fig. 10.3 The structure of mirtazapine.

Dose

The initial adult oral antidepressant dose is 15–30mg nocte. According to clinical response, this may be gradually increased over 2–4 weeks to a maximum of 45mg daily (taken either all as a bedtime dose or divided into 2 doses daily). Mirtazapine is not recommended for the treatment of depression in children and adolescents under the age of 18 years.

Side-effects

The commonest side-effects are:
- increased appetite
- weight gain
- drowsiness
- fatigue

- dizziness
- abnormal dreams
- insomnia
- dry mouth
- anxiety
- arthralgia
- oedema
- myalgia
- tremor
- confusion
- postural hypotension.

Less common side-effects include:
- mania
- hypotension
- hallucinations
- movement disorders.

Caution should be exercised in the following cases:
- elderly patients
- epilepsy or history of seizures
- hepatic impairment
- renal impairment
- cardiac disorders
- hypotension
- history of urinary retention
- susceptibility to angle-closure glaucoma
- diabetes mellitus
- psychosis
- history of bipolar depression.

Contraindications include:
- pregnancy
- breastfeeding.

Withdrawal should be gradual.

Reboxetine

This is a specific noradrenaline re-uptake inhibitor, or NARI for short.

Structure

The structure of reboxetine is shown in Fig. 10.4.

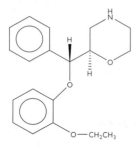

Fig. 10.4 The structure of reboxetine.

Dose

The initial adult oral antidepressant dose is 4mg twice daily (that is, a total daily dose of 8mg). According to clinical response, this may be increased after 3–4 weeks to 10mg daily, to be taken in divided doses. The maximum dose is 12mg daily (taken in divided doses). Reboxetine is not recommended for the treatment of depression in either children and adolescents under the age of 18 years or in elderly patients.

Side-effects

The commonest side-effects are:
- nausea
- anorexia
- insomnia
- headache
- sweating
- dizziness
- vasodilatation
- postural hypotension
- chills
- impotence
- urinary retention
- dry mouth
- difficulty with visual accommodation
- constipation
- tachycardia
- palpitations.

In elderly patients (for whom this drug is not recommended), reboxetine treatment may lower the plasma potassium ion concentration.

Caution should be exercised in the following cases:
- renal impairment
- hepatic impairment
- a history of epilepsy
- a history of cardiovascular disease
- bipolar disorder
- urinary retention
- prostatic hypertrophy
- susceptibility to angle-closure glaucoma.

Contraindications include:
- pregnancy
- breastfeeding.

Withdrawal should be gradual.

Venlafaxine

This serotonin and noradrenaline (norepinephrine) re-uptake inhibitor, or SNRI, was introduced into clinical practice in the UK in 1995.

℘ **Structure**

The structure of venlafaxine is shown in Fig. 10.5. It can be seen that it is not chemically related to the other antidepressant drugs described in this and previous chapters.

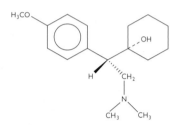

Fig. 10.5 The structure of venlafaxine.

♪ **Dose**

Before commencing pharmacotherapy with venlafaxine, it is important to carry out an ECG and to measure the blood pressure. These should then be carried out regularly during treatment; venlafaxine may cause prolongation of the QT interval, cardiac arrhythmias, tachycardia, and sustained hypertension.

The initial adult (>18 years) oral antidepressant dose is 37.5mg twice daily (that is, a total daily dose of 75mg). According to clinical response, this may be gradually increased to a maximum of 375mg daily, with each increment taking place at intervals of at least a fortnight. Venlafaxine is not recommended for the treatment of depression in children and adolescents under the age of 18 years.

A modified-release preparation is also available. The initial oral adult antidepressant dose of this modified-release preparation is 75mg daily, taken as one dose per day. According to clinical response, this may be increased after at least a fortnight to 150mg daily, again taken as one dose per day. The maximum dose of the modified release preparation is 375mg daily (again taken as one dose per day). The use of this modified release preparation is not recommended in children and adolescents under the age of 18 years.

The modified-release preparation may also be used for the treatment of generalized anxiety disorder and social anxiety disorder. The adult dose of this modified-release preparation is 75mg daily, taken as one dose per day. According to clinical response, the dose can be increased at intervals of at least a fortnight to a maximum of 225mg once daily. If there is no clinical benefit within 8 weeks, it may be best if this drug therapy is stopped. Again, the use of this modified release preparation is not recommended in children and adolescents under the age of 18 years.

☹ Side-effects

Side-effects include:

- generalized:
  - asthenia
  - chills
  - angio-oedema
- cardiovascular:
  - hypertension
  - vasodilatation (e.g. hot flushes)
  - palpitations
  - postural hypotension
  - arrhythmias
  - QT interval prolongation (rare)
- gastrointestinal:
  - decreased appetite
  - constipation
  - nausea
  - vomiting
  - bruxism
  - diarrhoea
  - gastrointestinal haemorrhage
- haematological/lymphatic:
  - ecchymosis
  - bleeding from mucous membranes
  - increased bleeding time
- metabolic/nutritional:
  - changes in serum cholesterol
  - weight loss
  - hyponatraemia
  - weight gain (perhaps less common than weight loss)
  - syndrome of inappropriate ADH secretion
- nervous system:
  - insomnia
  - abnormal dreams
  - nervousness
  - drowsiness
  - tremor
  - dizziness
  - headache
  - anxiety
  - hypertonia
  - confusional state
  - apathy
  - hallucinations
  - agitation
  - myoclonus
  - seizures (rare)
  - (hypo)mania (rare)
  - neuroleptic malignant syndrome (reported)
  - extrapyramidal side-effects (rare)

- incoordination
- aggression (rare)
- senses:
  - mydriasis
  - visual disturbances
  - visual accommodation abnormalities
  - changes in the perception of taste
  - tinnitus
  - angle-closure glaucoma (very rare)
- respiratory:
  - yawning
- dermatological:
  - rash
  - alopecia
  - photosensitivity
  - Stevens-Johnson syndrome (rare)
- urogenital:
  - decreased libido
  - erectile dysfunction
  - abnormal ejaculation
  - abnormal orgasm (more common in males)
  - anorgasmia
  - impaired micturition (e.g. hesitancy)
  - urinary retention
  - urinary incontinence (rare)
  - menorrhagia
- other:
  - dry mouth

Note that many of the warnings concerning withdrawal reactions and suicidal thoughts given in Chapter 9 in relation to the SSRIs also apply to venlafaxine. Withdrawal from treatment with this antidepressant should take place very gradually, under medical supervision.

As with tricyclic antidepressants, venlafaxine treatment may impair performance of skilled tasks such as operating machinery or driving. It is best to recommend to patients that they refrain from such activities while being treated with this drug.

Caution should be exercised in the following cases:
- heart disease
- diabetes mellitus
- history of epilepsy
- history of mania
- family history of mania
- susceptibility to angle-closure glaucoma
- concomitant use of drugs which prolong the bleeding time
- history of bleeding disorders
- hepatic impairment
- renal impairment.

Contraindications include:
- conditions associated with cardiac arrhythmia
- hypertension
- pregnancy
- breastfeeding.

Tryptophan

This amino acid (L-tryptophan) may be used as an adjunctive treatment for resistant depression, but should only be started under the supervision of an experienced specialist. Its use has been associated with the potentially fatal eosinophilia-myalgia syndrome.

Chapter 11

Treatment-resistant depression

Treatment-resistant depression *206*

Treatment-resistant depression

Although there is no generally accepted definition of treatment-resistant depression, NICE defines treatment-resistant depression as that which fails to respond to two or more antidepressants given sequentially at an adequate dose for an adequate time. David Christmas (2011) has published a particularly helpful algorithm to be used for the management of such treatment-refractory depression in primary care. The steps in this algorithm are as follows.

1. Lack of response?
2. If yes, then has a co-morbid diagnosis (such as anxiety disorder or substance misuse) been ruled out? If not, then review whether separate/additional treatment is required, which in many cases may be psychological.
3. If yes, then has the antidepressant dose been optimized and has the patient been taking it for an adequate duration? If not, then titrate to the maximum-tolerated dose and give this for either 6–8 weeks if there are no complicating factors, or for 10–12 weeks if co-morbid conditions are present.
4. If yes, then check whether the depressive episode has lasted for more than 2 years. If not, then consider the role of psychological therapy (if readily available).
5. If yes, then ensure that the patient has adequate exposure to psychological treatment approaches. Pharmacological options here include switching medications, or augmenting or combining medications.

Given its relatively mild side-effect profile and its unique mode of action, many might consider switching a treatment-resistant patient to agomelatine, which has been demonstrated to have efficacy in major depression. A difficulty with this option in the UK is that NICE have not given their appraisal of this new treatment. As Duerden (2011) explains:

'But there is no appraisal, and this is highly unlikely to appear in the next few years. Why is this? The explanation is that the drug company has decided not to submit evidence to NICE.

As stated on the NICE website, "The Appraisal Committee were due to meet on 23 June 2011 to discuss the use of agomelatine for the treatment of major depressive episodes. The manufacturer of agomelatine has informed NICE that they will not provide an evidence submission for this appraisal. Therefore, we are suspending the appraisal whilst we consider the next steps."

One next step is that NICE could do its own evidence review and health economic assessment, but this rarely happens presumably because it is labour intensive and the capacity to do this work is not available.'

Other drugs used in psychiatry

Benzodiazepines *208*
Non-benzodiazepine hypnotics *209*
Buspirone *210*
Beta-adrenoceptor blocking drugs *211*
Barbiturates *212*
Central nervous system stimulants *213*
Antimuscarinic drugs used in parkinsonism *214*
Drugs used in substance dependence *215*
Drugs for Alzheimer's disease *216*

Benzodiazepines

During the 1960s benzodiazepines were routinely used as hypnotics (e.g. nitrazepam and temazepam), and anxiolytics (e.g. diazepam and chlordiazepoxide). The Committee on Safety of Medicines have advised that benzodiazepines are indicated for the short-term relief of anxiety that is severe, disabling, or subjecting the individual to unacceptable distress. By short term, the Committee on Safety of Medicines mean a total time period of 2–4 weeks. They also advise that benzodiazepines should only be used to treat insomnia when it is severe, disabling, or causing extreme distress. Again, only short-term use should be made of benzodiazepines as hypnotics.

Since benzodiazepines may cause dependency, withdrawal needs to be gradual; a withdrawal syndrome may occur as long as 3 weeks after stopping the drug. Benzodiazepines also adversely impair the individual's ability to operate machinery or drive. They may also, paradoxically, cause increased aggression and hostility.

Non-benzodiazepine hypnotics

The following 3 newer hypnotics are less likely to cause dependency than benzodiazepines, and may be used for the short-term relief of insomnia:
• Zaleplon—very short acting; may be used for up to a fortnight.
• Zolpidem—short acting; may be used for up to a month.
• Zopiclone—short acting; may be used for up to a month.

Buspirone

This is an azaspirodecanedione which acts as a central 5-HT1A partial agonist and may be used in the short-term treatment of anxiety. Its main side-effects are dizziness, headache, light-headedness, excitement, and nausea.

Beta-adrenoceptor blocking drugs

Beta-blockers, such as propranolol, block peripheral beta-adrenergic receptors (for instance in the heart and peripheral vasculature). They are occasionally used in clinical psychiatric practice to treat anxiety symptoms, but do not help directly address the psychological symptoms of anxiety, such as fear.

Barbiturates

These are only extremely rarely used these days, e.g. to treat severe intractable insomnia in those patients who are already on such treatment.

Central nervous system stimulants

These are used mainly for the treatment of ADHD (or related hyperkinetic states) or sleep disorders (such as narcolepsy). They should be initiated only by specialists in child and adolescent psychiatry, in adult ADHD, or in sleep disorders.

Dexamfetamine is used to treat refractory ADHD and to treat narcolepsy. As an amfetamine (amphetamine), it may cause dependency, as well as many adverse side-effects.

Methylphenidate is used to treat ADHD and narcolepsy. Again, it is associated with many adverse side-effects.

Atomoxetine is a relatively newly introduced non-stimulant treatment for ADHD. Initially it was believed to be largely free of the adverse side-effects of psychostimulant medication for this disorder. However, it may be associated with potentially fatal hepatic disorders, albeit very rarely. Again, as with other treatments for ADHD, atomoxetine should be initiated only by an experienced expert specializing in the treatment of this disorder.

Modafinil is a newly-introduced central nervous system stimulant drug which is presently licensed for the treatment of daytime sleepiness associated with narcolepsy, obstructive sleep apnoea syndrome, and chronic shift work.

Antimuscarinic drugs used in parkinsonism

The drugs in this group include:
- procyclidine
- orphenadrine
- trihexyphenidyl (benzhexol).

These drugs tend to be used to offset the parkinsonian side-effects of antipsychotic drugs. However, these antimuscarinic drugs should not be routinely used with antipsychotic pharmacotherapy. One reason for this cautious approach is that not all patients being treated with antipsychotic drugs will necessarily develop parkinsonian side-effects. A second reason is that antimuscarinic drugs may give rise to antimuscarinic side-effects (as is only to be expected). Furthermore, antimuscarinic drugs may worsen tardive dyskinesia.

Drugs used in substance dependence

Under specialist supervision, the following classes of drugs may be used in the management of substance dependence:

- Benzodiazepines and clomethiazole—a reducing regimen may be used in managing alcohol withdrawal symptoms.
- Disulfiram—prophylactic adjunctive pharmacotherapy to prevent alcohol intake in alcohol dependence (by causing acetaldehyde to accumulate if alcohol is taken, leading to unpleasant systemic reactions).
- Acamprosate—this should be used in conjunction with counselling to help maintain abstinence in alcohol dependence.
- Methadone—a long-acting opioid agonist which can lessen withdrawal symptoms in opioid dependence by acting as a substitute for the opioid.
- Buprenorphine—used sublingually as an adjunct in managing opioid dependence.
- Lofexidine—used to lessen symptoms of opioid withdrawal.
- Naltrexone—this opioid-receptor antagonist is used to help prevent relapse in formerly opioid-dependent patients who are detoxified and have remained opioid-free for at least a week.

Drugs for Alzheimer's disease

In the UK, at the time of writing, the following 4 drugs are available for the treatment of Alzheimer's disease:

- donepezil
- galantamine
- rivastigmine
- memantine.

The first 3 of these are reversible inhibitors of acetylcholinesterase, while the 4th, memantine, is an NMDA (*N*-methyl-D-aspartate) antagonist. Initiation of treatment with these drugs should only be by a specialist with an expertise in the management of dementia, e.g. a consultant in old age psychiatry. The *British National Formulary* recommends that treatment with 1 of these 4 drugs should only continue 'if it is considered to have a worthwhile effect on cognitive, global, functional, or behavioural symptoms'.

References

Christmas D (2011). Recommended management of treatment-refractory depression. *Prescriber* **22**(21): 28–37.

Dorph-Petersen KA, Pierri JN, Perel JM, Sun Z, Sampson AR, and Lewis DA (2005). The influence of chronic exposure to antipsychotic medications on brain size before and after tissue fixation: a comparison of haloperidol and olanzapine in macaque monkeys. *Neuropsychopharmacology* **30**: 1649–61.

Duerden M (2011). Agomelatine: a new treatment for depression – but not NICE. *Prescriber* **22**(20): 7–8.

Fazel S, Grann M, and Goodwin GM (2006). Suicide trends in discharged patients with mood disorders: associations with selective serotonin reuptake inhibitors and comorbid substance misuse. *International Journal of Clinical Psychopharmacology* **21**: 111–15.

Gibbons RD, Hur K, Bhaumik DK, and Mann JJ (2005). The relationship between antidepressant medication use and rate of suicide. *Archives of General Psychiatry* **62**: 165–72.

Goldsmith L and Moncrieff J (2011). The psychoactive effects of antidepressants and their association with suicidality. *Current Drug Safety* **6**: 115–21.

Hale AS (1994). The importance of accidents in evaluating the cost of SSRIs: a review. *International Journal of Psychopharmacology* **9**: 195–201.

Healy D and Whitaker C (2003). Antidepressants and suicide: risk-benefit conundrums. *Journal of Psychiatry and Neuroscience* **28**: 331–7.

Ho BC, Andreasen NC, Ziebell S, Pierson R, and Magnotta V (2011). Long-term antipsychotic treatment and brain volumes: a longitudinal study of first-episode schizophrenia. *Archives of General Psychiatry* **68**: 128–37.

Isacsson G, Holmgren P, and Ahlner J (2005). Selective serotonin reuptake inhibitor antidepressants and the risk of suicide: a controlled forensic database study of 14,857 suicides. *Acta Psychiatrica Scandinavica* **111**: 286–90.

Jones PB, Barnes TR, Davies L, Dunn G, Lloyd H, Hayhurst KP, Murray RM, Markwick A, and Lewis SW (2006). Randomized controlled trial of the effect on Quality of Life of second- vs first-generation antipsychotic drugs in schizophrenia: Cost Utility of the Latest Antipsychotic Drugs in Schizophrenia Study (CUtLASS 1). *Archives of General Psychiatry* **63**: 1079–87.

Kirsch I (2009). Antidepressants and the placebo response. *Epidemiologia e Psichiatria Sociale* **18**: 318–22.

Konopaske GT, Dorph-Petersen KA, Sweet RA Pierri JN, Zhang W, Sampson AR, and Lewis DA (2008). Effect of chronic antipsychotic exposure on astrocyte and oligodendrocyte numbers in macaque monkeys. *Biological Psychiatry* **63**: 759–65.

Koo JY and Ng TC (2002). Psychotropic and neurotropic agents in dermatology: unapproved uses, dosages, or indications. *Clinics in Dermatology* **20**: 582–94.

Kuhn R (1958). The treatment of depressive states with G 22355 (imipramine hydrochloride). *American Journal of Psychiatry* **115**: 459–64.

Lieberman JA, Stroup TS, McEvoy JP, Swartz MS, Rosenheck RA, Perkins DO, Keefe RS, Davis SM, Davis CE, Lebowitz BD, Severe J, Hsiao JK; Clinical Antipsychotic Trials of Intervention Effectiveness (CATIE) Investigators (2005). Effectiveness of antipsychotic drugs in patients with chronic schizophrenia. *New England Journal of Medicine* **353**: 1209–23.

Maron E and Young AH (2011). Bipolar I disorder: current and future management options. *Future Prescriber* **12**: 14–18.

Martinez C, Rietbrock S, Wise L, Ashby D, Chick J, Moseley J, Evans S, and Gunnell D (2005). Antidepressant treatment and the risk of fatal and non-fatal self harm in first episode depression: nested case-control study. *British Medical Journal* **330**: 389.

Montgomery SA and Kasper S (2007). Severe depression and antidepressants: focus on a pooled analysis of placebo-controlled studies on agomelatine. *International Clinical Psychopharmacology* **22**: 283–91.

National Institute for Health and Clinical Excellence (2009). *Schizophrenia: Core interventions in the treatment and management of schizophrenia in adults in primary and secondary care*. NICE clinical guideline 82. NICE, London.

Owens DC (2011). Antipsychotics: is it time to end the generation game? *Prescriber* **22**(19): 48–50.

Puri BK (2011). Brain changes and antipsychotic medication. *Expert Review of Neurotherapeutics* **11**: 943–6.

Ramaekers JG (2003). Antidepressants and driver impairment: empirical evidence from a standard on-the-road test. *Journal of Clinical Psychiatry* **64**: 20–9.

Sansone RA and Sansone LA (2011). Agomelatine: a novel antidepressant. *Innovations in Clinical Neuroscience* **8**: 10–14.

Sherry RL, Rauw G, McKenna KF, Paetsch PR, Coutts RT, Baker GB (2000). Failure to detect amphetamine or 1-amino-3-phenylpropane in humans or rats receiving the MAO inhibitor tranylcypromine. *Journal of Affective Disorders* **61**: 23–9.

Watanabe N, Omori IM, Nakagawa A, Cipriani A, Barbui C, Churchill R, and Furukawa TA (2011). Mirtazapine versus other antidepressive agents for depression. *Cochrane Database of Systematic Reviews* **12**: CD006528. DOI: 10.1002/14651858.CD006528.pub2.

Whittington CJ, Kendall T, Fonagy P, Cottrell D, Cotgrove A, and Boddington E (2004). Selective serotonin reuptake inhibitors in childhood depression: systematic review of published versus unpublished data. *Lancet* **363**: 1341–5.

Index

A

absorption of drugs 14
acamprosate 7, 8, 215
acetylcholine 36
acute dystonic reactions 52
acute phase
  response 15–16
Addison's disease 7
ADHD 213
agomelatine 190–191, 206
agonists 32
akathisia 52
alcohol
  abuse-related liver
    disease 6–7
  drugs used in management
    of dependence 215
  enzyme induction 18
Alzheimer's disease 216
amisulpride 72–73
amitriptyline 138, 139,
  142–144
antagonists 32
antimanic drugs
  antipsychotics as 114
  asenapine 132–133
  benzodiazepines 114
  carbamazepine 122–126
  lithium salts 116–120
  quetiapine 130
  uses 114
  valproic acid 128–129
antimuscarinic effects 142
antimuscarinics 214
antipsychotic depot
  injections
  advantages and
    disadvantages 96
  buttock injection 96–98
  choice 101
  dosage guidelines 99
  equivalent doses 100
  flupentixol 102
  fluphenazine 103
  haloperidol 104
  lateral thigh
    injection 96–98
  olanzapine 105
  paliperidone 106
  pipotiazine 107
  risperidone 108
  site of injection 96–97
  timing 98
  z-track technique 98
  zuclopenthixol 109

antipsychotic drugs
  (non-depot)
  activities to avoid 48–49
  acute dystonic
    reactions 52
  akathisia 52
  amisulpride 72–73
  antimuscarinic
    interactions 214
  aripiprazole 74–75
  asenapine 93
  blood dyscrasias 48
  brain structure
    changes 56–57
  breastfeeding 48
  butyrophenones 41
  cardiovascular disease 48
  CATIE study 44
  cautions 48, 71
  chlorpromazine 60–61
  clozapine 76–79
  contraindications 49
  CUtLASS study 44
  dermatological use 38
  diphenylbuty-
    lpiperidines 41
  driving 48
  ECG recomm-
    endations 43, 46
  elderly 48, 58
  emergency
    administration 46
  epilepsy 48
  equivalent doses 45
  extrapyramidal
    symptoms 52–53
  first-generation
    (typical) 40–41
  flupentixol 66
  haloperidol 63
  high doses 46
  jaundice 48
  liver disease 8
  mania treatment 114
  neuroleptic malignant
    syndrome 54
  NICE recomm-
    endations 43
  non-psychotic uses 38
  olanzapine 80–83
  paliperidone 84–85
  parkinsonism 52–53
  Parkinson's disease 48
  perioral tremor 53
  phenothiazines 40
  photosensitization 49

pimozide 64–65
prostatic hypertrophy 48
quetiapine 86–89
rabbit syndrome 53
renal impairment 8
respiratory disease 48
risperidone 90–92
second-generation
  (atypical) 42, 71
substituted benzamides 41
sulpiride 41, 70
tardive dyskinesia 53
thioxanthenes 40–41
trifluoperazine 62
uses of 38
UV light exposure 49
withdrawal 50
zuclopenthixol
  (clopenthixol) 68–69
anxiolytics, liver disease 8
aripiprazole 74–75
asenapine 93, 132–133
assessment of patients 6–10
atomoxetine 8, 213
atypical antipsychotics 42,
  71

B

babies 30
barbiturates 18, 212
benzhexol 214
benzodiazepines
  alcohol withdrawal
    management 215
  driving and operating
    machinery 208
  hypnotic and anxiolytic
    use 208
  liver disease 8
  mania treatment 114
  withdrawal 208
beta-blockers 211
bioavailability 24
biotransformation 17–19
bipolar I disorder, treatment
  strategies 115
blood–brain barrier 16
blood–cerebrospinal fluid
  barrier 16
blood dyscrasias 48
brain structure,
  antipsychotic
  effects 56–57
breastfeeding 6, 48

buprenorphine 215
buspirone 8, 210
butyrophenones 41

C

Camcolit® 117
carbamazepine 8, 10, 18, 122–126
cardiovascular disease 48
carrier proteins 33
CATIE study 44
central nervous system stimulants 213
chlorpromazine 60–61
citalopram 184–185
classification of drugs 12
clearance 22–23
clomethiazole 215
clomipramine 148
clopenthixol, see zuclopenthixol
clozapine 9, 76–79
cognition 7
conjugation reactions 18
constant intravenous infusion 26–27
current medication 6
CUtLASS study 44
cycling processes 20
cyproterone acetate 7
cytochrome P450 monooxygenase system 18
cytochrome P450 polymorphisms 6
cytoplasmic second messengers 33

D

delusions 7
depot injections, see antipsychotic depot injections
dexamfetamine 213
diabetic patients, SSRI use 175
diagnostic hierarchy 4
diphenylbutylpiperidines 41
distribution of drugs 14–17
disulfiram 215
diuretics, interaction with SSRIs 175
divalproex sodium, see valproic acid
donepezil 216
dopamine 34
dosulepin 138, 139, 147
doxepin 151

driving 48, 141, 175, 202, 208
drug absorption 14
drug distribution 14–17
drug elimination 19–20
drug excretion 19–20
drug interactions 6
drug metabolism 17–19
drug receptors 32, 33
drug solubility 14
duloxetine 192–194
dyskinesias 52
dystonias 52

E

ECG 9, 43, 46, 64
ECT therapy 175
elderly
antipsychotic use 48, 58
pharmacokinetics 31
tricyclic antidepressant dose 137
electrocardiogram, see ECG
elimination of drugs 19–20
endocrinopathy 7
enteral administration 14
enterohepatic cycle 20
enzymes
induction 18
receptors as 33
epilepsy 48
escitalopram 8, 186–187
ethanol, see alcohol
excretion of drugs 19–20
extrapyramidal symptoms 52–53

F

family history 6
first-generation antipsychotics 40–41
first-order elimination 24
first-pass effect 18–19
first-pass elimination 19
first-pass metabolism 19
fluoxetine 8, 175, 178–179
flupentixol
antidepressant use 195
antipsychotic use (depot injection) 102
antipsychotic use (non-depot) 66
fluphenazine 19, 103
fluvoxamine 8, 177
food interactions, MAOIs 156–158
functional psychiatric disorders 3

G

G protein-coupled receptors 33
GABA 35
galantamine 216
gastric excretion 20
glomerular filtration 19
glutamate 35

H

haemodynamics 15
half-life 22, 23
haloperidol 63, 104
hepatic disease, drugs to avoid 7–8
herbal remedies 6
history taking 6–7
homicidal thoughts 7
hostility 7, 171
hydrolysis 18
hyperammonaemic encephalopathy 129
Hypericum perforatum 6
hyperprolactinaemia 61, 73
hypnotics
benzodiazepines 208
liver disease 8
non-benzodiazepine 209
renal impairment 8
hypoalbuminaemia 15
hypo-α₁-acid glycoproteinaemia 16

I

imipramine 19, 139, 145
insight 7
intravenous injection 24–25
inverse agonists 32
investigations 9–10
ion channels 33
isocarboxazid 164

J

jaundice 48
kidney
drug excretion by 19
drugs to avoid in kidney disease 8–9
Li-Liquid® 118
linear kinetics 24
lipid solubility 16
Liskonum® 117
lithium card 120
lithium
intoxication 118–119
lithium overdose 119

lithium salts 9, 10, 116–120
liver
  drug metabolism 17–19
  drugs to avoid in liver
    disease 7–8
lofepramine 138–139, 149
lofexidine 215

M

machinery operators 141,
  175, 202, 208
memantine 216
mental state examination 7
metabolism of drugs 17–19
methadone 215
methylphenidate 213
metoclopramide 41
mianserin 138, 153
mirtazapine 9, 196–197
moclobemide 166, 167–168
modafinil 8, 9, 213
monoamine-oxidase
  inhibitors (MAOIs)
  choice 159
  foods to avoid 156–158
  isocarboxazid 164
  liver disease 7
  medicines to
    avoid 156–158
  moclobemide 166,
    167–168
  over-the-counter products
    to avoid 156–158
  patient information
    cards 158
  phenelzine 161–163
  reversible (RIMAs) 166
  SSRI interactions 172
  tranylcypromine 159, 165
  tricyclic antidepressant
    interactions 156–158
  uses 156–158
  withdrawal 160
monoamine re-uptake
  inhibitors (MARIs) 142
multiple dosing 27–28

N

naltrexone 215
narcolepsy 213
National Institute for Health
  and Clinical Excellence
  (NICE) 43
needle phobics 7
neonates 30
neuroleptic malignant
  syndrome 54
neuroleptics, see
  antipsychotic drugs

neurotransmitter
  systems 34–36
NICE recommendations 43
noradrenaline
  (norepinephrine)
  34–35
noradrenaline
  re-uptake inhibitor
  (NARI) 198–199
nortriptyline 150
nuclear transcription
  regulating receptors 33

O

occupational history 6
olanzapine 9, 80–83, 105
one-compartment
  model 24–25
operating machinery 141,
  175, 202, 208
opioid dependence 215
organic psychiatric
  disorders 3
orphenadrine 214
over-the-counter
  medicines 6, 156–158
overdose
  lithium 119
  tricyclic antidepressants
    138–139
overvalued idea 7
oxidation 18

P

paediatric
  pharmacokinetics 30
paliperidone 84–85, 106
parenteral
  administration 14
parkinsonism 52–53, 214
Parkinson's disease,
  antipsychotic use 7, 48
paroxetine 173, 182–183
partial agonists 32
past medical history 6
patient information cards
  lithium therapy 120
  MAOIs 158
perioral tremor 53
pharmacokinetics 14–20
  absorption of drugs 14
  distribution of
    drugs 14–17
  elderly 31
  elimination of
    drugs 19–20
  metabolism of
    drugs 17–19

neonates and babies 30
terms and formulae 22–28
phase I and II
  metabolism 17–17–18
phenelzine 161–163
phenothiazines 18, 40
photosensitization 49
physical examination 7–9
pimozide 64–65
pipotiazine 107
placental drug
  transfer 16–17
plasma-protein
  binding 15–16
pregnancy 6, 16–17
presystemic elimination 19
presystemic metabolism 19
Priadel® liquid 118
Priadel® tablets 117
primary hypoadrenalism 7
procyclidine 214
prolonged QT interval 9,
  184, 186, 200
propranolol 211
prostatic hypertrophy 48
psychiatric disorders
  assessment of
    patients 6–10
  diagnostic hierarchy 4
  functional disorders 3
  non-pharmacological
    therapies 2
  organic disorders 3
  use of drugs 2
psychotropic drugs,
  classification 12

Q

QT prolongation 9, 184,
  186, 200
quetiapine 86–89, 130
Quicklet® 91

R

rabbit syndrome 53
rage 7
reboxetine 198–199
receptor superfamilies 33
reduction 18
renal excretion of
  drugs 19
renal impairment, drugs to
  avoid 8–9
respiratory disease 48
reversible
  monoamine-oxidase
  inhibitors (RIMAs) 166
risperidone 90–92, 108
rivastigmine 216

S

St John's wort 6
salivary excretion 20
saturation kinetics 24
second-generation (atypical)
    antipsychotics 42, 71
selective serotonin
    re-uptake inhibitors
    (SSRIs)
  cautions 175
  citalopram 184–185
  dependency 173
  diabetic patients 175
  diuretic interactions 175
  driving 175
  ECT therapy 175
  efficacy 176
  escitalopram 8, 186–187
  fluoxetine 8, 175,
    178–179
  fluvoxamine 8, 177
  hostility 171
  liver disease 8
  MAOI interactions 172
  operating machinery 175
  paroxetine 173, 182–183
  sertraline 9, 180–181
  side-effects 174–175
  suicide risk 171
  use 170
  venlafaxine 9, 173, 200–203
  withdrawal 173, 175
semisodium valproate,
    see valproic acid
Seroquel® XL 87–88, 89
serotonin 35
serotonin and noradrenaline
    re-uptake inhibitor
    (SNRI) 200–203
sertraline 9, 180–181
sodium valproate,
    see valproic acid
solubility of drugs 14
substance dependence 215
substituted benzamides 41
suicide risk 7, 171
sulpiride 41, 70
supplements 6

T

tardive dyskinesia 53
teratogenesis 17
tetracyclic
    antidepressants 138, 153
thioxanthenes 40–41
torsade de pointes 184, 186
total clearance 23
transmembrane non-enzyme
    receptors 33
transport proteins 33
tranylcypromine 159, 165
trazodone 152
treatment-resistant
    depression, 206
treatment-resistant
    schizophrenia 112
tricyclic (and related)
    antidepressant drugs
  amitriptyline 138, 139,
    142–144
  choice 138–139
  clomipramine 148
  dosage 137
  dosulepin 138, 139, 147
  doxepin 151
  driving 141
  elderly 137
  imipramine 19, 139, 145
  liver disease 8
  lofepramine 138–139,
    149
  MAOI interactions
    156–158
  nortriptyline 150
  operating machinery 141
  overdose 138–139
  sedative effects 138
  trazodone 152
  trimipramine 146
  uses 136
  withdrawal 140
trifluoperazine 62
trihexyphenidyl 214
trimipramine 146
tryptophan 204
two-compartment
    model 25

typical antipsychotics 40–41
tyramine-rich
    foods 156–158

U

UV light exposure 49

V

Valdoxan® (agomelatine)
    190–191, 206
valproate, see valproic
    acid
valproic acid 8, 9,
    128–129
Velotab® 81
venlafaxine 9, 173,
    200–203
vitamin D
    supplementation 129
volume of distribution 22

W

withdrawal
  antipsychotics 50
  benzodiazepines 208
  MAOIs 160
  SSRIs 173, 175
  tricyclic
    antidepressants 140

Z

z-track technique 98
zaleplon 8, 209
zero-order elimination 24
zolpidem 8, 209
zopiclone 8, 209
zuclopenthixol 68–69
zuclopenthixol acetate 68
zuclopenthixol
    decanoate 68, 109
zuclopenthixol
    dihydrochloride 68
Zydis® 81